OCT Made Easy

Edited by

Hiram G. Bezerra
Associate Professor of Medicine
Case Western School of Medicine
and
Director, Cardiac Catherization Laboratory
University Hospitals Cleveland Medical Center
Cleveland, Ohio

Guilherme F. Attizzani
Interventional Cardiology/Structural Heart Disease Intervention
Assistant Professor of Medicine and John C. Haugh Valve Fellow
Codirector, Cardiovascular Imaging Core Laboratory
Codirector, Valve and Structural Heart Disease Center
Harrington Heart and Vascular Institute
University Hospitals Cleveland Medical Center
Cleveland, Ohio

Marco A. Costa
Director, Interventional Cardiovascular Center
Director, Research and Innovation Center
Harrington Heart and Vascular Institute
University Hospitals Cleveland Medical Center
and
Professor of Medicine
Case Western Reserve University
Cleveland, Ohio

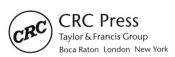
CRC Press
Taylor & Francis Group
Boca Raton London New York

CRC Press is an imprint of the
Taylor & Francis Group, an **informa** business

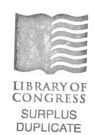

CRC Press
Taylor & Francis Group
6000 Broken Sound Parkway NW, Suite 300
Boca Raton, FL 33487-2742

Printed and bound in India by Replika Press Pvt. Ltd.

Printed on acid-free paper

International Standard Book Number-13: 978-1-4987-1456-3 (Paperback)

**Visit the Taylor & Francis Web site at
http://www.taylorandfrancis.com**

**and the CRC Press Web site at
http://www.crcpress.com**

OCT Made Easy

Contents

Contributors   ix

1. Optical coherence tomography imaging for stent planning   1
Daniel Chamié and Emile Mehanna
1.1   Introduction   1
1.2   General outline   2
1.3   Preintervention OCT imaging   3
1.4   Postintervention OCT imaging   14
1.5   Potential clinical impact of OCT use for PCI planning and guidance   21
References   23

2. OCT imaging for assessment of plaque modification   29
Ruben Ramos and Lino Patrício
2.1   Introduction   29
2.2   Plain ordinary balloon and drug-eluting balloon angioplasty   29
References   42

3. OCT for plaque modification   43
Andrejs Erglis
3.1   Plaque modification before coronary artery stenting using cutting/scoring balloon   43
3.2   Cutting and scoring balloons   43
3.3   Trial results with cutting or scoring balloon plaque pretreatment   45
3.4   Patient's clinical cases using cutting and scoring plaque pretreatment   46
References   58

4. OCT for stent optimization   59
Satoko Tahara, Yusuke Fujino, and Sunao Nakamura
4.1   Introduction   59
4.2   Utilization of OCT for vessel preparation   59
4.3   OCT for defining stent length and diameter   60
4.4   OCT for side branch protection   64
4.5   Conclusion   72
References   72

5. OCT for left main assessment   75
Yusuke Fujino
5.1   Introduction   75
5.2   Safety of FD-OCT for ULM Disease   75
5.3   FD-OCT Measurements for ULM Disease   77
5.4   Feasibility of FD-OCT for ULM Disease   78
5.5   Conclusions   82
References   82

6. Optical coherence tomography for late stent failure   85
Tej Sheth, Anthony Fung, and Catalin Toma
6.1   Introduction   85
6.2   Restenosis   85
6.3   Case report: In-stent restenosis   89
6.4   Stent thrombosis   91
References   94

7. OCT assessment in spontaneous coronary artery dissection   97
Christopher Franco, Lim Eng, and Jacqueline Saw
7.1   Spontaneous coronary artery dissection   97
7.2   Role of OCT in the diagnosis and management of spontaneous coronary artery dissection   102
7.3   Management of SCAD   105
7.4   Future directions   107
7.5   Conclusions   107
References   107

8. Optical coherence tomography assessment for cardiac allograft vasculopathy after heart transplantation   111
Sameer J. Khandhar and Guilherme Oliveira
8.1   Introduction   111
8.2   Screening and diagnosing CAV   112
8.3   CAV Pathophysiology   112
8.4   OCT utilization post–heart transplantation   115
8.5   Treatment of CAV   119
8.6   Conclusion   119
References   119

9. OCT assessment out of the coronary arteries   **123**
Jun Li, Daniel Kendrick, Vikram S. Kashyap, and Sahil A. Parikh

9.1   Introduction   123
9.2   History of intravascular imaging   123
9.3   Optical coherence tomography   124
9.4   Clinical applications of OCT in the peripheral vasculature   126
9.5   Future directions   132
References   133

10. Optical coherence tomography for the assessment of bioresorbable vascular scaffolds   **135**
Yohei Ohno, Alessio La Manna, and Corrado Tamburino

10.1   Introduction   135
10.2   Optical coherence tomography assessment before BVS implantation   136
10.3   Optical coherence tomography assessment after BVS implantation   138
10.4   Optical coherence tomography assessment for BVS follow-up   139
Disclosures   142
References   142

11. ILUMIEN OPTIS Mobile and OPTIS Integrated Technology Overview   **145**
Tsung-Han Tsai and Desmond Adler

11.1   Platform overview   145
11.2   ILUMIEN OPTIS Mobile System   148
11.3   OPTIS Integrated System   150
11.4   OCT application software   155
11.5   Angio coregistration software   158
11.6   Conclusion   160
References   160

12. Terumo OFDI system   **163**
Kenji Kaneko, Tetsuya Fusazaki, and Takayuki Okamura

12.1   Introduction   163
12.2   FastView imaging catheter   163
12.3   LUNAWAVE OFDI imaging console   166
12.4   Case report: Usefulness of OFDI-guided PCI for the separated proximal and mid–left anterior descending artery lesions   172
     Tetsuya Fusazaki
12.5   Case report: Usefulness of 3D OFDI for bifurcation PCI   177
     Takayuki Okamura
Videos   179
Acknowledgment   179
Disclosures   179
References   180

13. **OCT imaging acquisition** 181

Manabu Kashiwagi, Takashi Kubo, Hironori Kitabata, and Takashi Akasaka

13.1 Introduction 181
13.2 System of OCT 181
13.3 Imaging procedure 182
13.4 Flushing parameters: Recommended injection setting 183
13.5 Pitfalls and limitations 183
13.6 Conclusions 187
References 187

Appendix: Intravascular bioresorbable vascular scaffold optimization technique 189
Jun Li and Hiram Bezerra

Index 197

Contributors

Desmond Adler
St. Jude Medical, Inc.
St. Paul, Minnesota

Takashi Akasaka
Professor
Department of Cardiovascular Medicine
Wakayama Medical University
Wakayama, Japan

Daniel Chamié
Interventional Cardiologist
Invasive Cardiology Department
Dante Pazzanese Institute of Cardiology
and
Director
Optical Coherence Tomography Core Laboratory
Cardiovascular Research Center
São Paulo, Brazil

Lim Eng
Cardiology Fellow
Division of Cardiology
Vancouver General Hospital
and
Department of Medicine
University of British Columbia
Vancouver, Canada

Andrejs Erglis
Professor of Medicine and Chief
Latvian Centre of Cardiology
Pauls Stradins Clinical University Hospital
and
Director
Institute of Cardiology and Regenerative Medicine
University of Latvia
Riga, Latvia

Christopher Franco
Cardiology Fellow
Division of Cardiology
Vancouver General Hospital
and
Department of Medicine
University of British Columbia
Vancouver, Canada

Yusuke Fujino
Interventional Unit
Cardiovascular Department
New Tokyo Hospital
Matsudo, Japan

Anthony Fung
Clinical Professor
Division of Cardiology
Vancouver General Hospital
and
University of British Columbia
Vancouver, Canada

Tetsuya Fusazaki
Associate Professor
Division of Cardiology
Department of Internal Medicine and Memorial
Heart Center
Iwate Medical University School of Medicine
Morioka, Japan

Kenji Kaneko
Project Manager
Interventional Systems Division
Cardiac and Vascular Company
Terumo Corporation
Tokyo, Japan

Manabu Kashiwagi
Research Associate
Department of Cardiovascular Medicine
Wakayama Medical University
Wakayama, Japan

Vikram S. Kashyap
Professor of Surgery
Case Western Reserve
University School of Medicine
and
Chief
Division of Vascular Surgery and Endovascular
Therapy
and
Co-Chair
Clinical Executive Committee
Harrington Heart and Vascular Institute
University Hospitals Cleveland Medical Center
Cleveland, Ohio

Daniel Kendrick
Vascular Surgery Fellow
Department of Surgery
Case Western Reserve University School of Medicine
and
Division of Vascular Surgery and Endovascular
Therapy
Harrington Heart and Vascular Institute
University Hospitals Cleveland Medical Center
Cleveland, Ohio

Sameer J. Khandhar
Assistant Professor of Clinical Medicine
Department of Cardiology
Perelman School of Medicine
University of Pennsylvania
and
Heart and Vascular Institute at Penn-Presbyterian
Hospital
Philadelphia, Pennsylvania

Hironori Kitabata
Assistant Professor
Department of Cardiovascular Medicine
Wakayama Medical University
Wakayama, Japan

Takashi Kubo
Assistant Professor
Department of Cardiovascular Medicine
Wakayama Medical University
Wakayama, Japan

Alessio La Manna
Consultant Interventional Cardiologist
Department of Cardiology
Ferrarotto Hospital
University of Catania
Catania, Italy

Jun Li
Interventional Cardiology Fellow
Department of Medicine
Case Western Reserve University School of Medicine
and
Department of Interventional Cardiology
Division of Cardiovascular Medicine
Harrington Heart and Vascular Institute
University Hospitals Cleveland Medical Center
Cleveland, Ohio

Emile Mehanna
Cardiology Fellow
Department of Internal Medicine
Division of Cardiology
Harrington Heart and Vascular Institute
University Hospitals Case Medical Center
and
Case Western Reserve University
Cleveland, Ohio

Sunao Nakamura
Interventional Unit
Cardiovascular Department
New Tokyo Hospital
Matsudo, Japan

Yohei Ohno
Assistant Professor
Department of Cardiology
Ferrarotto Hospital
University of Catania
Catania, Italy
and
Department of Cardiology
Tokai University School of Medicine
Isehara, Japan

Takayuki Okamura
Associate Professor
Division of Cardiology
Department of Medicine and Clinical Science
Yamaguchi University Graduate School of Medicine
Ube, Japan

Guilherme Oliveira
Harrington Heart and Vascular Institute
University Hospitals Case Medical Center
Case Western Reserve School of Medicine
Cleveland, Ohio

Sahil A. Parikh
Director of Endovascular Services
Center for Interventional Vascular Therapy
Division of Cardiology
Department of Medicine
Columbia University Medical Center
New York–Presbyterian Hospital
New York, New York

Lino Patrício
Consultant
Cardiology Department
Hospital de Santa Marta
Centro Hospitalar Lisboa Central
Lisbon, Portugal

Ruben Ramos
Consultant
Cardiology Department
Hospital Santa Marta
and
Centro Hospitalar de Lisboa Central
Lisbon, Portugal

Jacqueline Saw
Clinical Professor
Division of Cardiology
Vancouver General Hospital
and
Department of Medicine
University of British Columbia
Vancouver, Canada

Tej Sheth
Associate Professor of Medicine
McMaster University
Population Health Research Institute
Hamilton Health Sciences
Hamilton, Canada

Satoko Tahara
Interventional Unit
Cardiovascular Department
New Tokyo Hospital
Matsudo, Japan

Corrado Tamburino
Professor
Department of Cardiology
Ferrarotto Hospital
University of Catania
and
Excellence Through Newest Advances (ETNA)
Foundation
Catania, Italy

Catalin Toma
Assistant Professor of Medicine
Director, Interventional Cardiology
Heart and Vascular Institute
University of Pittsburgh Medical Center
Pittsburgh, Pennsylvania

Tsung-Han Tsai
St. Jude Medical, Inc.
St. Paul, Minnesota

Chapter 1

Optical coherence tomography imaging for stent planning

Daniel Chamié and Emile Mehanna

1.1 INTRODUCTION

Since its introduction in 1977, percutaneous coronary intervention (PCI) has undergone continued and profound advancements. The evolution of coronary devices, operator's experience, interventional techniques, and adjunctive pharmacotherapy dramatically reduced the risks of early complications and improved long-term outcomes, elevating PCI to the predominant modality of invasive treatment of coronary artery disease (CAD) and one of the most frequently performed therapeutic interventions in medicine.[1]

Although coronary angiography is the mainstay imaging modality to assess the presence, extent, and severity of CAD, and to guide PCI procedures, intravascular imaging has played a fundamental role during PCI maturation and evolution. Visual estimation of the planar silhouette of the contrast-filled luminogram may be insufficient for accurate diagnosis of CAD severity and extension, and oftentimes does not allow accurate planning and optimization of PCI. By providing higher-resolution tomographic images of the entire circumference of the vessel wall, intracoronary imaging may overcome these limitations.

In the mid-1990s—when coronary stents were plagued by elevated rates of acute or subacute thrombosis, and oral anticoagulants were part of the adjunctive pharmacotherapy with its associated hemorrhagic complications—Colombo et al.[2] demonstrated that despite an optimal angiographic result (<20% residual stenosis), only 30% of the stents implanted in 420 lesions were adequately expanded by intravascular ultrasound (IVUS). After IVUS-guided high-pressure balloon postdilatation, full expansion and complete stent apposition were achieved in 96% of the patients. This strategy resulted in very low rates of acute (0.6%) and subacute (0.3%) stent thrombosis, eliminating the need for systemic anticoagulants, and consolidating the widespread use of coronary stents for the percutaneous treatment of CAD in the years to come.

Over the last two decades, IVUS guidance helped reduce the rates of restenosis and repeat revascularization after bare-metal stents—but not myocardial infarction (MI) and mortality. Despite the absence of adequately powered randomized trials to demonstrate whether routine IVUS guidance improves clinical outcomes after drug-eluting stent (DES) implantation, four contemporary meta-analyses suggest that IVUS guidance can reduce stent thrombosis, MI, repeat revascularization, and mortality when compared with angiographic DES guidance alone.[3–6]

Despite these benefits, and after more than 20 years of clinical use, IVUS has been used in less than 20% of PCI procedures.[7]

More recently introduced, optical coherence tomography (OCT) uses near-infrared light to generate cross-sectional images of the coronary arteries. Near-infrared light has a shorter wavelength and higher frequency than ultrasound, thus providing images with 10-fold higher resolution than those provided by IVUS. The faster and safe acquisition of longitudinal sequences of sharp and detailed images, along with ease of use and interpretation, leverages OCT as an attractive imaging modality with the potential to guide and optimize PCI, which ultimately may translate into improved clinical outcomes.

In this chapter, we discuss the usefulness of OCT in planning and guiding coronary stenting, using a practical, case-oriented approach, whenever applicable.

1.2   GENERAL OUTLINE

Although at first sight the term *stent planning* may be viewed as a synonym for *stent guidance*, the two concepts are not always applied interchangeably. When it comes to the use of adjunctive intravascular imaging with the intention to guide coronary interventions, it is common practice to perform PCI based on angiography, and only execute intravascular imaging at the end of the procedure, to check the "final" PCI result. Although this approach offers the opportunity to optimize PCI, the planning strategy has been overlooked and restricted to the inherent limitations of angiography. As so, it is our opinion that the use of intravascular imaging for stent planning carries a much broader role, and intravascular imaging pre-PCI should not be underestimated.

Intravascular OCT pre-PCI allows accurate quantification of stenosis severity and extension, and characterization of the underlying plaque components and morphometry, helps locate adequate landing zones for the stent to be implanted, and provides accurate vessel sizing for selection of the stent length and diameter. It also allows up-front anticipation of the need for balloon postdilatation and the type and size of the balloon to be used. In other words, stent optimization can also be planned based on pre-PCI OCT imaging. After a satisfactory angiographic result has been achieved, post-PCI OCT can be performed to check on the procedure results, and judge whether further iterations are still needed.

Based on the concepts outlined above, we give pre-PCI imaging equal or higher importance than post-PCI imaging. As so, this chapter is presented according to the following structure:

- Preintervention OCT imaging
  - Basic nomenclature and definitions
  - Assessment of coronary stenosis severity
  - Assessment of lesion morphology, composition, and morphometry
  - Vessel measurements for stent sizing
- Postintervention OCT imaging
  - Verification and optimization of stent expansion
  - Verification and optimization of stent apposition
  - Assessment of other qualitative parameters after stenting (edge dissection, tissue prolapse, and in-stent thrombus formation)

1.3 PREINTERVENTION OCT IMAGING

1.3.1 Assessment of coronary stenosis severity

1.3.1.1 Basic nomenclature and definitions

According to the Consensus Standards for Acquisition, Measurement, and Reporting of Intravascular Optical Coherence Tomography Studies document,[8] the magnitude and extension of coronary lumen compromise by a stenosis rely on determination of the minimal lumen area (MLA) within the stenosis, and percent of lumen stenosis relative to the vessel references, leading to the following definitions:

- *Stenosis*: Lesion with at least 50% compromise of its lumen cross-sectional area in comparison with a predefined reference segment lumen.
- *MLA*: Lesion site with the smallest lumen area measurement.
- *Distal reference*: Site with the largest lumen distal to a stenosis, within the same segment, with no major intervening branches; this may not be the site with the least plaque.
- *Proximal reference*: Site with the largest lumen proximal to a stenosis, within the same segment, with no major intervening branches; this may not be the site with the least plaque.
- *Lumen area stenosis*: (Reference lumen area − Minimum lumen area within the lesion)/Reference lumen area. For lumen area stenosis calculation, the reference segment used can be the distal, proximal, smallest, largest, or average of the distal and proximal references.
- *Lesion length*: Distance between the distal and proximal references.

The sharper delineation of the lumen–wall interface, coupled with smooth longitudinal lumen visualization, enables automatic lumen segmentation over the entire vessel length imaged by current Fourier-domain OCT (FD-OCT) systems, generating a volumetric lumen profiling and three-dimensional rendering that includes the lesion and its adjacent reference segments, with all pertinent quantifications. The MLA and its diameter and area stenosis are automatically calculated. This volumetric lumen profiling capability can be of great utility to assist operators in the catheterization laboratory in identifying adequate vessel references and properly sizing the target vessel for appropriate device selection. Figure 1.1 exemplifies the quantification of coronary artery stenosis severity by OCT.

1.3.1.2 Considerations of quantitative measurements of vascular structures

Due to inherent differences in resolution, wavelength, and scattering properties of light and sound, measurements taken by OCT and IVUS are expected to be different. In fact, when analyzing the same anatomic structure, IVUS measurements are known to be consistently larger than those provided by OCT.[9–11] With the previous generation of time-domain OCT (TD-OCT)—which required proximal vessel occlusion for transitory blood clearance during image acquisition—these differences were mostly attributed to possible reductions in coronary perfusion pressure that could lead to partial vessel collapse, with smaller measures made by OCT.[9–11]

Lumen areas measured by IVUS have been reported to be as large as 33.7% relative to TD-OCT with occlusion techniques for image acquisition, and 21.5% larger when compared with nonocclusive techniques.[11]

Smaller differences have been described between IVUS and the current FD-OCT systems.[12–14] FD-OCT systems have a faster image acquisition rate, allowing blood clearance to be accomplished by transient contrast media flush through the guiding catheter during fast imaging catheter pullbacks, without the need for vessel occlusion. In addition, the FD-OCT imaging catheter size is similar to the IVUS catheter size, such

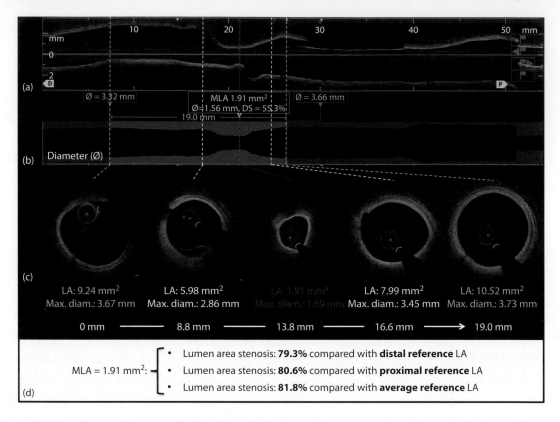

Figure 1.1 Identification of anatomic landmarks and calculation of stenosis severity. (a) Longitudinal view of an OCT pullback obtained distal (left) to proximal (right) across a mid–left anterior descendent artery (LAD) lesion. (b) Volumetric lumen profile feature present in the current FD-OCT system, Ilumien Optis (St. Jude Medical, St. Paul, Minnesota). (c) Selected cross section images from the locations indicated by vertical bars on the longitudinal and lumen profile views. The dashed red bar indicates the site with the MLA. The cross sections with the largest lumen areas distal and proximal to the MLA site (dashed blue bars) represent the distal and proximal references, respectively. Lesion length is easily determined by measuring the distance between the distal and proximal reference sites. Lumen area stenosis can be determined by comparing the MLA against the distal reference lumen area, the proximal reference lumen area, or the average of the distal and proximal reference lumen areas (d). Of note, the automatic lumen segmentation throughout the entire OCT pullback allows the generation of a lumen profile map of the entire vessel length. The MLA is automatically identified, and possible references offered by the algorithm. By adjusting one or either references on the lumen profile tool, the lesion length is automatically adjusted and the MLA site updated, together with automatic calculation of the stenosis severity (diameter or area stenosis).

that the degree of coronary pressure reduction and vessel collapse due to the presence of the imaging catheter is thought to be comparable between both imaging modalities. Therefore, any lumen measurement difference between FD-OCT and IVUS is not likely to be associated with the imaging procedure itself, but with the fundamental physical differences and resolutions between the two methods.

To address this issue, Kubo et al.[14] investigated the differences and accuracy of lumen quantification among angiography, IVUS, and FD-OCT in a multicenter study that included 100 patients with CAD. Compared with FD-OCT, quantitative coronary angiography (QCA) measured smaller (relative difference –5%) and IVUS measured larger (relative difference 9%) minimal lumen diameters (MLDs). Likewise,

IVUS measurements of MLA were 10% higher than those obtained by FD-OCT ($p < 0.001$). Importantly, interobserver variations of IVUS measurements were twice as high as those of OCT (root mean square deviation 0.32 mm^2 vs. 0.16 mm^2). In an additional analysis of five phantom models of known lumen dimensions (lumen diameter 3.08 mm, lumen area 7.45 mm^2), lumen areas measured by FD-OCT were equal to the actual lumen area of the phantom models, while IVUS overestimated the true lumen area by 8% ($p < 0.001$ vs. FD-OCT). The higher accuracy and reproducibility of OCT for quantification of lumen dimensions was confirmed in other *in vitro* and *in vivo* studies.[12,15–17]

1.3.1.3 Estimating the functional significance of coronary stenoses by quantitative OCT measurements

The first step in the planning strategy starts with identifying the stenosis that will benefit from revascularization. Having in mind the measurement differences between IVUS and OCT, clinicians should refrain from applying IVUS-derived parameters to define coronary stenosis severity to OCT studies.

Over the years, it became common practice to use anatomic parameters derived from IVUS to estimate the functional significance of angiographically intermediate (40%–70%) coronary stenoses. A variety of observational studies validated IVUS-derived parameters against invasive and noninvasive tests for the assessment of lesion severity. However, low sensitivities (66.3%–92%), specificities (56%–92%), and positive predictive values (27%–67%), as well as poor accuracy (64%–72%), limit the clinical application of such parameters for predicting the physiological significance of coronary stenoses.

Due to more accurate and reproducible lumen quantification, it was expected that OCT could provide better diagnostic efficiency in identifying hemodynamically severe coronary stenoses. At present, six studies have compared OCT-derived parameters with fractional flow reserve (FFR) for intermediate lesion assessment (Table 1.1).[18–23] As expected, the MLA cutoff values that better predicted an FFR of <0.80 were significantly smaller than those traditionally used for IVUS, ranging from 1.59 to 2.88 mm^2. Although OCT slightly improved sensitivity (75%–93.5%), specificity (63%–90%), and positive predictive value (66%–80.6%) in comparison with previous IVUS data, this intravascular imaging showed only moderate efficiency to determine functionally significant lesions, with accuracy ranging from 72% to 87%. These data reinforce the low specificities of intravascular anatomic metrics to predict functionally significant stenosis, precluding the routine use of intravascular imaging tools as substitutes for functional evaluation for decision making of intermediate angiographic stenoses.

1.3.2 Assessment of lesion morphology, composition, and morphometry

In the pre-PCI planning, qualitative lesion assessment allows better understanding of the disease pathophysiology, adding complementary information to the clinical decision making, as well as the identification of features that would be associated with worse acute results of interventional procedures.

A profound discussion on plaque characterization is beyond the scope of this chapter and is described elsewhere. Various animal and human postmortem validation studies have demonstrated that OCT can differentiate among fibrous, lipidic, and calcific components of atherosclerotic plaques with high sensitivity and specificity.[24–26]

OCT also allows precise identification and quantification of high-risk features associated with plaque instability and vulnerability, such as the presence of lipid and its longitudinal and circumferential distribution, the quantification of fibrous cap thickness (an important predictor of plaque rupture),[27,28] and macrophage infiltration (a marker of intraplaque inflammation).[29,30] In comparison with other imaging modalities, such as IVUS and angioscopy, OCT showed higher accuracy and sensitivity in identifying plaque rupture, dissection, erosion,

TABLE 1.1
OCT MLA cutoffs to predict functionally significant nonleft main intermediate stenoses as determined by FFR

	N	OCT System	FFR Cutoff	MLA Cutoff	AUC	Sensitivity	Specificity	PPV	NPV	Accuracy
Gonzalo et al. (2012)[18]	61	FD	0.80	1.95	0.74	82%	63%	66%	80%	72%
Shiono et al. (2012)[19]	62	TD	0.75	1.91	0.90	93.5%	77.4%	80.6%	92.3%	85.4%
Reith et al. (2013)[20]	62	FD	0.80	1.59	0.81	75.8%	79.3%	80.6%	74.2%	77.4%
Pawlowski et al. (2013)[21]	71	TD[a]	0.80	2.05	0.91	75%	90%	70.6%	92.6%	87%
Pyxaras et al. (2013)[22]	55	FD	0.80	2.88	0.78	73%	71%	N/A	N/A	72%
Reith et al. (2015)[23]	142 (all lesions)	FD	0.80	1.64	0.83	78.8%	75.8%	80.8%	73.4%	N/A
	80 (diabetics)	FD	0.80	1.59	0.84	76.6%	78.8%	83.7%	70.3%	N/A
	62 (nondiabetics)	FD	0.80	1.64	0.83	78.8%	75.9%	78.8%	75.9%	N/A

Note: AUC, area under the receiver operating characteristic curve; N/A, not available; NPV, negative predictive value; PPV, positive predictive value.

[a] Nonocclusive technique used with the TD-OCT technology.

calcified nodules, and intracoronary thrombus,[31] which may be of particular importance in the evaluation of acute coronary syndrome (ACS) patients. The capability of differentiating predominantly red from predominantly white thrombus adds some insights into estimating the timing of the occurrence of the acute event.[32]

OCT studies have shown that patients presenting with ST-elevation myocardial infarction (STEMI) had significantly thinner fibrous caps protecting the lipid or necrotic core than patients presenting with non-ST-elevation myocardial infarction (NSTEMI) or stable angina.[33,34] Fibrous cap thickness was thinner in patients presenting with resting angina in comparison with those presenting with exercise-induced angina.[35] Thin-cap fibroatheroma (TCFA), plaque rupture, and red thrombus are more frequent in STEMI patients than in NSTE ACS and stable patients.[34] ACS patients presenting with preserved protective fibrous caps were shown to have better prognoses than those presenting with plaque rupture.[36] When plaque rupture is present, it has been shown that a "proximal-type" rupture of the fibrous cap is more often seen in STEMI patients, while "distal-type" apertures are more frequent in patients with NSTEMI.[34] Detailed qualitative and morphometric assessments of atherosclerotic plaques, in combination with quantitative measures, provide important pathophysiological and prognostic information that may be of value during the clinical decision-making process, and may assist physicians in individualizing management. Figures 1.2 and 1.3 illustrate situations where high-resolution quantitative and morphometric information of the underlying plaque helped the clinical decision making.

Although coronary stents have minimized the impact of lesion morphology on the acute and chronic results of PCI compared with balloon angioplasty, some morphologic features are still of contemporary importance. Severe coronary calcification limits stent expansion, which can be associated with adverse events, including restenosis and stent thrombosis. It is important to acknowledge that severely calcified lesions—especially in small vessels or very stenotic lesions—are hard to cross, and the preintervention imaging may not be feasible. However, whenever imaging is possible, accurate recognition and quantification of coronary calcium may allow for refinements in the initial interventional strategy and implementation of plaque modification strategies (e.g., atheroablation and scoring balloons). Aspects to consider are the circumferential arc of calcium and its longitudinal length, axial thickness, and proximity to the lumen.[37] Treating stent underexpansion in a heavily calcified lesion is more difficult than preventing it.[38] This may be of particular importance with the recent introduction of polymeric bioresorbable scaffolds, a technology less forgiving of overexpansion and excessive high-pressure balloon dilatation than metallic stents (Figure 1.4).

Conversely, TCFA, as determined by OCT, has been identified as a predictor for periprocedural complications. In a study by Tanaka et al., the presence of lipid-rich plaques with an overlying fibrous cap thickness of ≤65 μm was identified as an independent predictor of no reflow after successful stenting in patients with NSTE ACS. The frequency of no reflow increased significantly, and the final thrombolysis in myocardial infarction (TIMI) myocardial blush grade deteriorated according to the amplitude of the lipid arc in the culprit plaque.[39]

In a study of 115 ACS patients successfully treated with stenting, culprit lesions were classified in three groups according to the pre-PCI findings: (1) ruptured plaque (*n* = 59), (2) nonruptured TCFA (*n* = 21), and (3) nonruptured, non-TCFA (*n* = 35). Nonruptured TCFAs (43%) were significantly more often associated with microvascular obstruction as determined by cardiac contrast-enhanced magnetic resonance imaging than ruptured plaques (27%) and nonruptured, non-TCFA plaques (9%). Interestingly, the prevalence of microvascular obstruction increased as the fibrous cap thickness decreased.[40] Following the same pathophysiological principles, TCFA was also identified as an independent predictor for type IVa (periprocedural) MI.[41,42] Lastly, the presence of TCFA at the stent landing zone is responsible for a sixfold increase in the risk of having a stent edge dissection.[43]

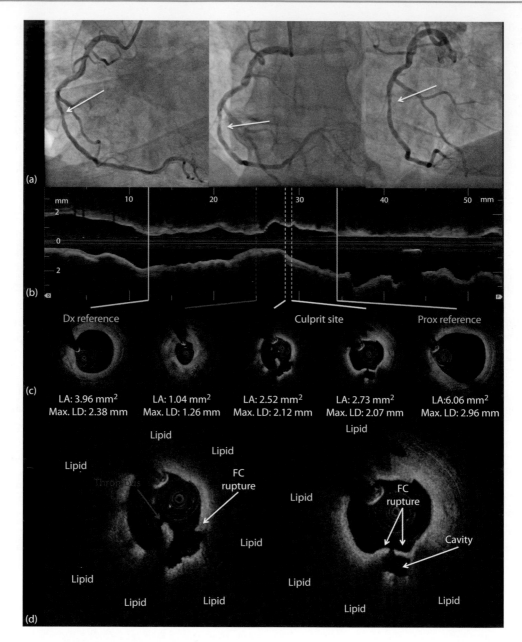

Figure 1.2 A 58-year old diabetic patient was referred to cardiac catheterization 4 days after an inferior wall STEMI. He had been managed by intravenous fibrinolytics within 2 hours of the symptoms' onset, and achieved clinical and electrocardiographic signs of reperfusion, being asymptomatic since then. His coronary angiography revealed a single, intermediate (52% diameter stenosis by QCA) lesion in the mid–right coronary artery (RCA) (a). Global left ventricular function was preserved, with mild inferomedial hypokinesia. (b) Longitudinal view of an OCT pullback, with corresponding cross section images of key vascular sites (c). The MLA site (lumen area 1.04 mm²) is predominantly fibrotic, promoting a severe (79.2% lumen area stenosis) stenosis in comparison with the average of distal (Dx) and proximal (Prox) lesion references. The culprit site is located proximal to the MLA region, at the so-called "plaque shoulder" (zoomed cross sections in panel d). The underlying plaque is predominantly lipid-rich with a minimum fibrous cap (FC) thickness of 50 µm. The site of plaque rupture is clearly visible, with an empty cavity and some remnants of intraluminal thrombus. This lesion was eventually treated with a DES implantation guided by OCT.

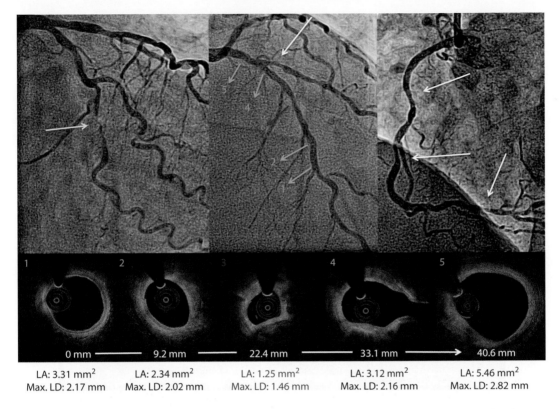

Figure 1.3 **Top panel presents angiographic images of a 64-year-old female diabetic patient, who presented with exertional angina of recent onset (over the past 4 months) and a positive treadmill stress test.** Apart from the subtotal lesion in the second obtuse marginal branch of the left circumflex artery, intermediate (50%–70%) stenoses were observed in the left anterior descendent artery (LAD), first diagonal branch, and right coronary artery, adding up a Syntax score of 28. Her surgical risk was low (EuroSCORE II 0.94%, Society of Thoracic Surgeons [STS] score 0.67%). Invasive physiological assessment of the right coronary artery (RCA) (FFR = 0.82) and first diagonal branch (FFR = 0.85) ruled out the presence of myocardial ischemia in the territories supplied by these vessels. The FFR measurement of the LAD was 0.80 after two measurements with 140 and 180 µg/Kg/min of continuous intravenous infusion of adenosine. OCT (bottom panel) evaluation revealed a long (40.6 mm) segment of atherosclerotic disease composed primarily of fibrocalcific plaques. The MLA was 1.25 mm², generating a lumen area stenosis of 71.6%. Due to the stable plaque phenotype and a borderline FFR, the decision was to treat the OM2 lesion only and maintain the patient under optimal medical treatment. After discharge, she resumed normal activities, and started exercising. After 13 months, the patient is still asymptomatic with no ischemia detected in a maximum treadmill test and perfusion myocardial scintigraphy.

1.3.3 Vessel measurements for stent sizing

The selection of devices of adequate diameters (to match the target vessel dimensions and maximize the final stent area achieved) and lengths (to cover the entire target lesion) is crucial to successful acute and long-term outcomes of PCI.

1.3.3.1 *Length measurement*

Precise length measurement is important to provide coverage of the entire target lesion and to avoid coverage of undesirable regions. OCT images are acquired with automated pullbacks that may reach

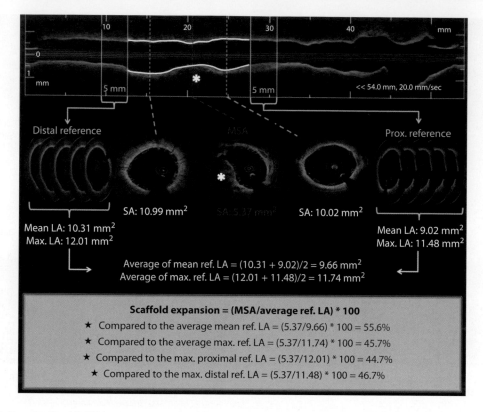

Figure 1.4 Longitudinal OCT image (top panel) and corresponding cross section images after implantation of a polymeric bioresorbable scaffold in a calcified coronary lesion without proper predilatation. Note the eccentric scaffold expansion (middle cross section image) at the site of a very superficial and thick calcified plaque. Despite its minimum scaffold area of above 5.0 mm², the expansion at this site is only 45.7% of what was expected according to the average lumen area of the distal and proximal references. Significant scaffold underexpansion irrespective of the expansion criteria used. Had this plaque been better evaluated, preventive measures could have been adopted to prevent such scaffold underexpansion.

out to 40 mm/s. A faster pullback speed provides more accurate and reproducible length measurements, devoid of cardiac and respiratory motion artifacts.[44] Importantly, length measurements are not possible with manual catheter pullback.

Lesion length—which will dictate stent length—is determined as the distance between the distal and proximal references. Slightly different concepts are used for reference identification when using IVUS and OCT. In addition to looking at lumen dimensions, operators also take into consideration the quantification of plaque burden in the search for the vessel references when using IVUS. An IVUS study showed residual plaque burden at stent edges to be a predictor of stent edge restenosis. A plaque burden cutoff of 47% best separated edge restenosis from no restenosis—although with only moderate discriminatory ability (*c*-statistic 0.69). Due to the limited penetration of light into the vessel wall, and depending on the plaque thickness and composition, vessel external elastic membrane (EEM) may not be visible by OCT. As a consequence, plaque burden may not be quantified. Thus, reference sites by OCT are defined as the regions with the largest lumen dimensions proximal and distal to a stenosis, within the same segment, with no major intervening branches.[8] Importantly, this may not be the site with the least plaque burden.

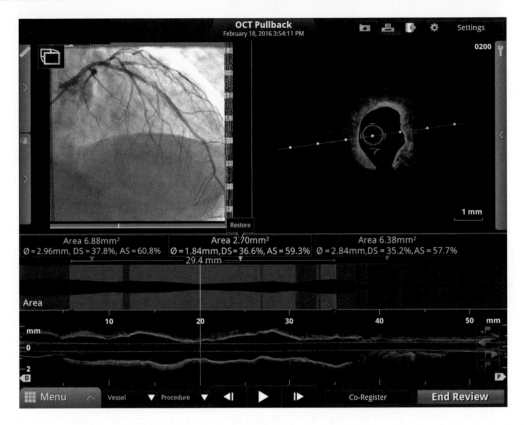

Figure 1.5 The integrated OPTIS© software (St. Jude Medical, St. Paul, Minnesota), allowing simultaneous display of coregistered angiographic images (white marker in the top left image) with corresponding OCT cross-sectional images (top right) and longitudinal luminal profile display with online measurements of lesion and reference vessel parameters.

Some of the reasons OCT operators are less concerned about plaque burden at the vessel references are as follows. Although plaque burden indicates the magnitude of plaque buildup, it reflects poorly the degree of lumen stenosis. According to the Glagov phenomenon, positive remodeling of the diseased arterial wall compensates the accumulation of atherosclerotic plaque, ultimately preserving lumen dimensions. This is well illustrated in a study of 884 patients submitted to coronary intervention, where only 6.8% of the angiographically "normal" references were free of disease by IVUS. Of note, the average plaque burden of angiographically normal (nonstenosed) references was 51 ± 13%.[45] Due to the higher resolution of OCT, one would expect to see even more disease at apparently normal angiographic references. Furthermore, in the setting of complex and diffuse atherosclerotic disease (where intravascular imaging may play a more decisive role), identification of regions with small plaque burden may be a challenge and misleading. In this situation, one should seek the regions with the largest lumen dimensions proximal and distal to the target stenosis, irrespective of the plaque burden behind. Conversely, when the EEM is visible by OCT, distal and/or proximal to the stenosis, it is an indication of a less diseased vessel, and appropriate "normal-looking" references can be more easily identified.

The composition and morphometry of underlying atherosclerosis at the site of the intended stent landing zone may be of greater importance than the plaque burden alone to predict risks of complications after stenting. In an analysis of 395 stent edges, our group demonstrated that in addition to the presence of atherosclerotic disease at the stent landing zone, circumferential calcium angle, fibrous cap thickness, and presence of TCFA at the stent edges were also independent predictors for edge dissections. A minimum fibrous cap thickness of ≤80 μm was the best cutoff to predict a dissection when the stent border was placed over a lipid-rich plaque with a sensitivity and specificity of 73.9% and 72.5%, respectively. When a TCFA was present at the stent edge, the odds of having a dissection were 6.16 (95% confidence interval [CI] 1.42–26.69, p = 0.016). Calcified plaques were frequently observed in dissected stent edges (40.6%), and their circumferential extension was identified as an independent predictor of dissection (odds ratio [OR] 1.02 for every 1° increase; 95% CI 1.00–1.03, p = 0.017). A calcium angle of ≥72° was identified as the best cutoff to predict calcium-related edge dissections with a sensitivity of 71.1% and specificity of 71.2%. Interestingly, the calcium depth relative to the lumen surface was not associated with the occurrence of edge dissections, suggesting that loss of circumferential vessel compliance might be more important in the pathogenesis of calcium-related edge dissections rather than the presence or depth of calcium.[43]

One obvious, but not less important consideration, is the need to coregister the sites selected on OCT and on angiography, making sure the stent positioning under fluoroscopy is aligned to the sites previously measured by OCT. The current FD-OCT system synchronizes the highly detailed OCT images with angiography, making coregistration between both imaging methods accurate, easier and intuitive with the potential to minimize positioning errors during the procedure (Figure 1.5).

1.3.3.2 Diameter measurement

There are a number of options to size the stent diameter by OCT. Typical measurements, from the least to most aggressive, are as follows (Figure 1.6):

- Maximum lumen diameter of the smallest reference
- Average of the maximum lumen diameter of both references
- Maximum lumen diameter of the largest reference
- Mean diameter from midwall to midwall (between lumen and media)
- Mean diameter from media to media

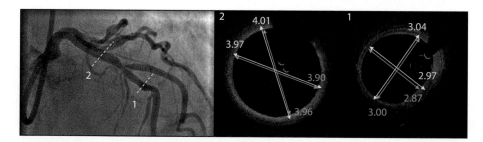

Figure 1.6 Options of diameter measurements for stent sizing. The left panel shows an angiography image of a left anterior descendent artery (LAD)/D1 lesion. The LAD distal and proximal references are indicated by the numbers 1 and 2, respectively. The right panel presents OCT cross section images correspondent to the references indicated on angiography. Lumen diameter measurements are in green, and the EEM diameter measurements are in yellow.

The consistently smaller (though, more accurate) measures of vascular dimensions by OCT in comparison to IVUS, together with the limited visualization of the EEM (true vessel size) by OCT, led to recent concerns that OCT-guided stent sizing would lead to inappropriate stent expansion.

In a small, single-center study, Habara et al.[46] randomized 70 patients with *de novo* coronary lesions to OCT- versus IVUS-guided stenting. In either group, the opposite imaging method was performed after the final result was deemed acceptable by the imaging method assigned by randomization. In the OCT group, final stent expansion was assessed by IVUS, while in the IVUS group, final stent apposition was assessed by OCT. Despite the interesting design, the authors did not acknowledge the inherent differences between IVUS and OCT and used the same guidance protocol for both imaging modalities—a large flaw of the study. Good visibility of the vessel wall was defined as visualization of ≥270° of the EEM circumference. References were located according to the ability of the imaging methods to visualize the EEM both distal and proximal to the lesion, and sites with plaque burden <50% were selected. At these regions, the largest lumen areas were used for sizing the stent diameter, and the distance between the proximal and distal references determined the stent length. When the EEM was not visible, reference sites and stent length were determined by angiography. Stent deployment pressure was determined by measuring the EEM at the MLA site; when this was not possible, stents were deployed according to angiography. After stenting, postdilatation was performed if (i) residual plaque burden at the MSA site was >50%; (ii) MSA was <90% of the distal reference lumen area, and (iii) incomplete stent apposition was seen. When the EEM was not seen at the lesion site, the need for postdilatation and the balloon size were based on angiography. As expected, EEM was seen in >270° of the vessel circumference by OCT in 62.9% of the distal and proximal edges, but only in 8.6% at the MSA site. Conversely, IVUS was able to visualize the EEM at the distal and proximal edges in 100% of the cases, and at the MSA site in 94.3% ($p < 0.001$, for all comparisons). Thus, by the adopted protocol, stent sizing (diameter and length) and optimization in the OCT group were in fact performed according to angiographic parameters in approximately 40% and 90% of the cases, respectively. Consequently, in the OCT group stents were deployed with lower pressures (9.8 ± 2.4 atm vs. 14.2 ± 3.4 atm, $p < 0.001$), postdilatation was less frequently performed (60% vs. 85.7%, $p = 0.03$), and postdilatation pressures were smaller (13.5 ± 3.4 atm vs. 16.1 ± 4.7 atm, $p = 0.03$) than in the IVUS group. As a result, this inappropriate OCT guidance protocol resulted in smaller stent expansion in comparison to IVUS guidance (64.7 ± 13.7% vs. 80.3 ± 13.4%, $p = 0.002$), with higher frequency of residual reference segment stenosis at the proximal edge (plaque burden: 42.2% vs. 36.5%, $p = 0.02$).

In the ILUMIEN II study, Maehara et al.[47] compared OCT-measured stent dimensions after OCT guidance from the ILUMIEN I study ($n = 354$) with IVUS-measured stent dimensions after IVUS guidance from the ADAPT-DES study ($n = 586$). By correctly acknowledging that IVUS measurements are known to be larger than OCT measurements, the authors did not use absolute MSA for a valid cross-study comparison. The percent of stent area expansion (MSA relative to the reference lumen area) was used instead. This is a *post hoc* comparison of two different studies, and therefore, randomization is absent. Although covariate-adjusted analysis and propensity score matching were performed, unmeasured confounders could not be ruled out. Additionally, standardized imaging protocols were not utilized in both studies. Of note, for the entire population, the prevalence of preintervention imaging was 57.7% for IVUS and 93.7% for OCT ($p < 0.0001$). In the matched-pair analysis ($n = 240$ pairs), the degree of stent expansion was not significantly different between OCT and IVUS guidance (median [first, third interquartiles] = 72.9% [63.3, 81.3] vs. 70.6% [62.3, 78.8], $p = 0.29$). After adjustment for baseline differences in the entire population ($n = 940$), the degree of stent expansion was also not different between the two imaging methods ($p = 0.84$). As discussed previously, pre-PCI imaging is of great importance for PCI planning, and it can affect stent sizing and its final expansion. This step was largely overlooked in the IVUS group included in the ILUMIEN II study.

More recently, the ILUMIEN III study randomized 450 patients in a 1:1:1 fashion to angio-guided (n = 146), IVUS-guided (n = 146), and OCT-guided (n = 158) PCI. In this study, a specific protocol was used for OCT-guided stent sizing: when the EEM was seen in at least 180° of the vessel circumference, the mean EEM diameter was measured in both the distal and proximal references, and the smaller of these diameters, rounded down to the nearest 0.25 mm, was used to determine the stent diameter. If the EEM was not visible, the smallest mean lumen diameter was used instead. The postdilation balloon could be no larger than the nearest reference vessel EEM diameter, or up to 0.5-mm larger than the post-PCI mean reference lumen diameter (if the EEM was not visible). By following this specific protocol, the primary endpoint of post-PCI minimum stent area was not significantly different between OCT-guided and IVUS-guided PCI (5.79 mm² vs. 5.89 mm², p = 0.42). No significant differences were observed in respect to the minimum (87.6% vs. 86.5%, p = 0.77) and mean stent expansion (105.8% vs. 106.3%, p = 0.63). OCT-guided procedures resulted in similar minimum stent areas (5.79 mm² vs. 5.49 mm², p = 0.12), but higher minimum (87.6% vs. 82.9%, p = 0.02) and mean stent expansion (105.8% vs. 101.4%, p = 0.001) when compared to angiography-guided PCI.[48]

The following suggestions are based on the authors' experience, and may differ among other operators. Whenever the EEM is visible in 180° to 270° of both references, we use the mean EEAM diameter for stent sizing. If the EEM is not visible, we use the maximum lumen diameter of the largest reference instead. In cases with significant vessel tapering, we use the mean EEM diameter (when seen in 180° to 270° of the vessel circumference) or the maximum lumen diameter (if the EEM is visible in less than 180° of the vessel circumference) of the smaller reference. In this situation, the selected stent will be smaller than the largest reference, and thus, postdilatation with noncompliant balloons sized according to the largest reference diameter is recommended to accomplish adequate expansion and apposition throughout the entire treated length. An example of OCT-guided stent sizing and tailored postdilatation according to the information derived from the pre-PCI imaging is presented in Figure 1.7.

1.4   POSTINTERVENTION OCT IMAGING

The main goal of PCI is to eliminate myocardial ischemia by optimizing the gain of lumen dimensions without complications. Ideally, the implanted stent should be symmetrically expanded, with final lumen dimensions that match the reference vessel dimensions, and should be completely apposed to the vessel wall, with no edge dissections. In this regard, adequate strategy planning and device sizing by pre-PCI imaging does not ensure that a good and optimized result will always be achieved. Intravascular imaging post-PCI allows the operator to verify the success of the initially planned strategy, and to further plan the next approaches to optimize and maximize the stent implantation within the safety margins of the target vessel. Thus, post-PCI imaging should be viewed as complementary to pre-PCI imaging. The role of OCT to assess the quality of stent implantation and optimize the PCI results will be discussed in the sections to come.

1.4.1   Verification and optimization of stent expansion

Stent underexpansion has long been identified as an important predictor of early stent thrombosis and mid- to long-term in-stent restenosis (ISR) of both bare-metal stent (BMS) and DES.[49–65]

Stent expansion has been traditionally determined by comparing the minimal stent area with the reference lumen area. Because there are many possible reference measurements, several approaches exist for the quantification of stent expansion. The reference segment used can be the distal, proximal, or average of the

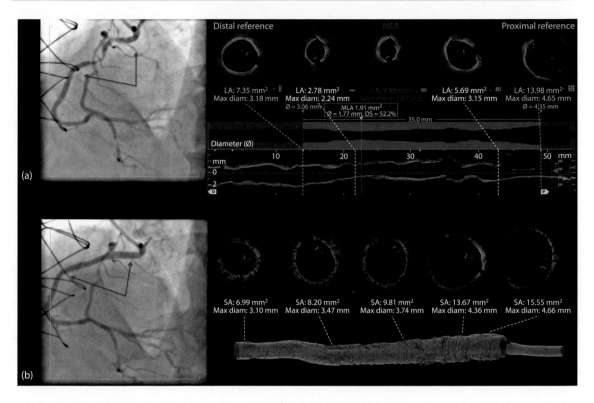

Figure 1.7 OCT use for stent sizing. (a) Angiography of a long and severe lesion in the proximal right coronary artery. OCT was performed after predilatation with a 2.0 × 20 mm noncompliant balloon and administration of 200 μg of intracoronary nitroglycerin. The longitudinal OCT view, lumen profiling, and selected cross section images along the diseased segment are presented. The distal and proximal references were selected by identification of the largest lumen area both distal and proximal to the MLA region. The distance between these reference regions measured 35 mm. Of note, the EEM was visible in more than 180° of vessel circumference in both references, indicating adequate targets for stent landing. Important vessel tapering was seen between the proximal (maximum LD 4.65 mm) and distal (maximum LD 3.18 mm) references. Thus, using the maximum diameter of the largest reference would impose an increased risk of injury to the distal vessel reference. On the other hand, it would be difficult to make a 3.0 mm stent (sized according to the distal reference) match the proximal vessel reference. Thus, by knowing the exact vessel measurements throughout the target segment, our strategy was to (1) implant a 3.5 × 38 mm DES deployed with low pressure (6 atm) to avoid injury to the distal edge, (2) use postdilatation with a 3.5 × 20 mm noncompliant balloon with progressively increasing pressure from distal to proximal (maximal inflation pressure 30 atm), (3) use focal postdilatation with a 4.5 × 15 mm noncompliant balloon targeted only at the proximal stent segment, and (4) perform poststenting OCT to check on the stent expansion and apposition and look for signs of potentially harmful complications. The postintervention angiography and OCT results are presented in panel b. Note that adequate stent expansion and apposition were achieved, with a progressive increase in stent dimensions from distal to proximal, respecting the natural vessel tapering. The anatomic restoration of the vessel lumen postintervention is confirmed by three-dimensional OCT reconstruction of the lumen surface, presented in the bottom panel. No further iterations were needed after the postintervention OCT.

distal and proximal references. Additionally, the average of either all lumen areas or the maximum lumen areas at each reference have been used for comparison. As a result, a single standardized criterion has never been established, and certainly would not apply for all anatomies. Thus, it is important to specify what criterion is being used for the assessment of stent expansion. In Figure 1.4, one can find an example of stent expansion assessment according to different comparator standards.

Previous IVUS studies have investigated several different criteria to define an optimal stent expansion that would be associated with freedom from major adverse cardiac events. Various post-PCI MSA cut points have been proposed as thresholds to predict BMS (around 6.5 mm^2) and DES (ranging from 5.0 to 5.7 mm^2) failure.[56,58,60,63,66]

Due to the differences between IVUS and OCT measurements, one should be cautious in translating previously validated IVUS criteria to OCT examinations. In a large (900 lesions treated with 1001 stents in 786 patients) and multicenter registry, Soeda et al. identified, in an exploratory analysis, OCT-derived MSA values of 5.0 mm^2 for DES and 5.6 mm^2 for BMS as the best cutoffs to predict device-oriented cardiac events. As expected, these cutoffs are slightly smaller than those identified in previous IVUS studies. However, the positive predictive values of these OCT-derived metrics were very low (5.6% for DES and 17.5% for BMS), limiting their ability to discriminate device-oriented cardiac events. Conversely, the negative predictive values were high (97.8% for DES and 92.7% for BMS), suggesting that final OCT-derived MSAs greater than these thresholds could be associated with low rates of 1-year adverse events. Importantly, a single absolute value of MSA is not applicable to all vessel sizes, may not apply to stents deployed in tapered vessels, and does not allow the perception of multiple sites of underexpansion along the treated segment. Additionally, 21.7% of the cases were performed with the previous-generation TD-OCT system—already removed from clinical practice—which is known to provide smaller measurements than the current FD-OCT. The degree to which the MSA cutoffs were contaminated by the TD-OCT measurements was not measured. Finally, the low 1-year event rate of 4.5%, mostly driven by target lesion revascularizations, may also limit the ability of such cutoffs to predict more meaningful hard endpoints (e.g., death, MI, and stent thrombosis).

Thus, dedicated OCT-derived criteria to determine optimal stent implantation that would be associated with good clinical outcomes need to be created and validated in properly designed and powered studies. Investigators do not necessarily need to revalidate already established IVUS criteria. The ability of current OCT technology to dispose high-quality images with high sampling rates (180 frames/s) and high-speed pullbacks (up to 40 mm/s), devoid of major artifacts, enables accurate three-dimensional rendering of the stent and vessel wall. As a result, in addition to the eye-catching beautiful images, OCT has the potential to shift the assessment of stent expansion postimplantation from single area measurement cut points to a more comprehensive and volumetric assessment of global stent geometry.

1.4.2   Verification and optimization of stent apposition

It is imperative to understand the conceptual differences between stent expansion and apposition. While expansion refers to the final stent area relative to a predefined reference lumen area, apposition refers to the contact of the stent struts with the vessel wall. It is thus perceivable that the two terms are not interchangeable, and may occur in isolation or coexist.

Stent malapposition (or ISA) is defined as separation of the stent struts from the vessel lumen wall in a region not overlying a side branch. By both IVUS and OCT, ISA is expressed at the cross section level as area. When intravascular imaging is acquired with motorized pullbacks, the longitudinal length of ISA can be easily determined. Factoring multiple ISA areas over a specific stent length will enable the calculation of ISA volume. The higher axial resolution of OCT, in combination with a lumen environment clear from blood, further expanded the evaluation of ISA down to the strut level, enabling assessment of the apposition status of every imaged strut with high sensitivity and accuracy. Detailed descriptions of cross section and strut-level quantification of ISA are given elsewhere.

Temporally, ISA can be classified as (1) acute, identified immediately after the stenting procedure; (2) persistent, identified after the index procedure, and still visible at follow-up evaluations; and (3) late acquired, not present postprocedure, but detected at follow-up assessment. Based on this temporal classification, it is intuitive to note that not all ISAs share the same pathophysiology, and do not portend the same prognostic impact. Acute ISA is usually related to procedural factors (e.g., mismatch between stent and vessel size, uneven stent expansion, plaque-related factors, lumen irregularities, and eccentricity), while late-acquired ISA can result from late positive vascular remodeling not compensated by abluminal tissue growth, plaque regression, or thrombus dissolution behind the stent struts without vessel remodeling,[67–70] etc. Over time, acute ISA can fully resolve (complete vascular healing), reduce in size (unfinished vascular healing), remain stable, or increase in size (plaque regression and positive remodeling).

While late-acquired ISA may be associated with late DES thrombosis[71–79]—especially ISA in the setting of positive remodeling,[80] or with large malapposition areas[81] or frank aneurysm formation[82]—acute ISA (provided the stent is well expanded) has not been consistently related to adverse events.[62,63,77,83,84]

The incidence of acute ISA on OCT studies ranges from 13% to 65% on a lesion-based analysis, and from 0.6% to 7.5% on a strut-level analysis.[47,75,79,85–88] Acute ISA size and strut-to-lumen distances have been identified as independent predictors for ISA persistence and delayed vascular healing.

A large OCT study detected acute ISA in 62% of 356 lesions in 351 patients—50% of which were located at stent edges—and measured 1.16 ± 0.69 mm^2. Thirty-one percent of the acute ISA persisted over 28.6 ± 10.3 months, but decreased in size to 0.88 ± 0.71 mm^2. Edge location and ISA volume were independent predictors for ISA persistence. An ISA volume of >2.56 mm^3 best differentiated persistent from resolved ISA.[79]

An OCT study of 66 different stent designs in 43 patients identified 78 segments of acute ISA in 36 patients. After 6 months, 71.5% of the ISA segments had completely healed. ISA volume and maximum strut-to-lumen distance were independent predictors of ISA persistence and delayed healing. Of note, all struts with maximum ISA distances of <270 µm after stent implantation were completely apposed and covered by tissue at 6 months. On the other hand, ISA distances of ≥850 µm resulted in persistent ISA and grossly delayed coverage in 100% of the cases.[89] A similar strut-to-lumen distance cutoff (≤260 µm) was identified in another study to best separate resolved from persistent malapposed struts (sensitivity 89.3%, specificity 83.7%, area under the curve 0.884) after first-generation DES implantation.[87] More recently, a strut-to-lumen distance of ≤380 µm was identified as the best cutoff to predict resolved strut ISA in everolimus-eluting stents (sensitivity 93.5%, specificity 69.8%, and area under the curve 0.878).[90]

In a computational fluid dynamics simulation, Foin et al.[91] characterized flow profile and shear stress distribution of different cases of ISA with increasing strut-to-wall distances, ranging from 100 to 500 µm. Protruding (but apposed struts) and struts with moderate detachment (ISA detachment distance of <100 µm) sowed minimal blood flow disturbance compared with floating struts with larger detachment distances. The *in vivo* impact of these ISA distance thresholds was assessed in a retrospective OCT analysis of 72 stents (48 patients) serially at baseline and at 6-month follow-up. In line with previous reports, this study confirmed the association of ISA distance and incomplete strut coverage at follow-up. Acute malapposed segments with a strut-to-vessel distance of <100 µm showed complete coverage at 6 months, whereas the rate of uncovered struts increased from 6.1% with ISA distances of 100 and 300 µm to 15.7% with ISA distances of >300 µm.

The clinical impact of such ISA distance thresholds is uncertain, and the magnitude of acute malappositions that should be corrected by further balloon dilatation is still an open question. At present, it seems reasonable to proceed with additional balloon dilatation, adjusted to the lumen dimension at the maximum ISA region, to correct grossly large and longitudinally long malappositions (Figure 1.8).

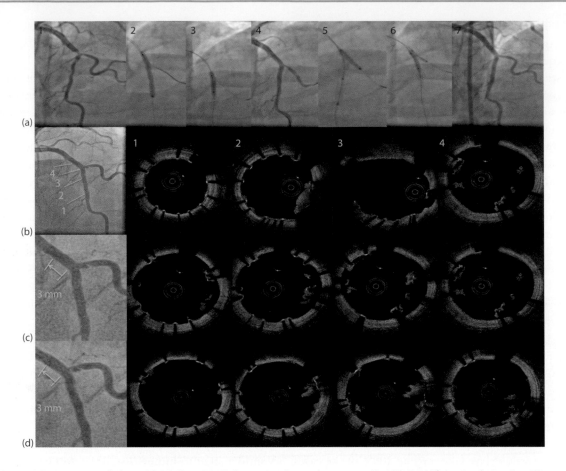

Figure 1.8 Acute stent failure. (a) Medina 1:1:1 left anterior descendent artery (LAD)/D2 bifurcation lesion in a 59-year-old man presenting with stable angina Canadian Cardiovascular Society (CCS) 3 (1). A 3.0 × 30 mm DES was implanted (2) and postdilated with a noncompliant 3.0 × 15 mm balloon throughout its entire length (3). Side branch pinching was noted in the control angio (4), dilated with a noncompliant 2.5 × 12 mm balloon (5), and final kissing balloon inflation was performed (6). (7) Satisfactory final angiographic result. The patient was discharged the next day, and remained asymptomatic until the 27th day post-PCI, when he presented to a primary care facility with anterior wall STEMI, managed with early administration of tenecteplase. Clinical and electrocardiographic signs of reperfusion were achieved, and the patient was referred to cardiac catheterization 7 days after the acute event (b). The angiography revealed no stenosis with preserved TIMI 3 flow, unchanged in comparison with the final angiography taken at the index PCI. OCT examination revealed adequate expansion and apposition along the entire stent segment distal to the bifurcation (1 and 2), with signs of residual intraluminal thrombus (2) (four and five o'clock). No struts were seen overhanging the side branch ostium (3), while a large stent malapposition was seen throughout the stent segment proximal to the bifurcation, with residual thrombus attached to the malapposed struts (4). (c) Consecutive OCT cross sections of the 3 mm segment of stent malapposition proximal to the bifurcation. At the site of maximum malapposition, the lumen area was 10.1 mm^2 and the stent area was only 5.9 mm^2, resulting in a malapposition area (4.2 mm^2) almost as large as the stent area. The maximum strut-to-lumen distance measured 880 μm. (d) OCT cross sections matched to the ones presented in panel c after dilatation of the proximal stent segment with a 4.0 × 6 mm semicompliant balloon. Note the complete resolution of the stent malapposition. Although acute malapposition has not been consistently associated with adverse cardiac events, it seems reasonable to proceed with additional balloon dilatation to correct grossly large malappositions, particularly when affecting a long consecutive segment of the stent.

1.4.3 Assessment of other qualitative parameters after stenting

1.4.3.1 Stent edge dissections

Stent edge dissections are characterized by unplanned vessel tearing that occurs at the transition between the rigid stent cage and the adjacent arterial wall—a region of compliance mismatch. Edge dissections are defined as disruptions of the arterial lumen surface in the stent edge segments (either 5 mm proximal or distal to the stent borders).[43,92] Their incidence ranges widely from 20% to 56%.[41,43,47,85–87,92–95] Stent borders positioned over diseased reference segments (particularly with eccentric plaques), certain plaque types (e.g., calcified, lipid-rich, and TCFA), morphometry at the stent landing zone (e.g., calcium angle and fibrous cap thickness), stent and lumen eccentricity, and mismatches between stent and lumen dimensions have been identified as key predictors for stent edge dissections.[43] The vast majority (84%) of the OCT-detected edge dissections are not apparent on angiography,[43] have a favorable healing profile over the course of 6–9 months,[85–87,93,94] and are not associated with adverse clinical events at 1 year.[43,85,87,95] Thus, while unpleasant to the eyes, operators should refrain from implanting additional stents to treat small, non-flow-limiting edge dissections that are only visible by OCT (Figure 1.9).

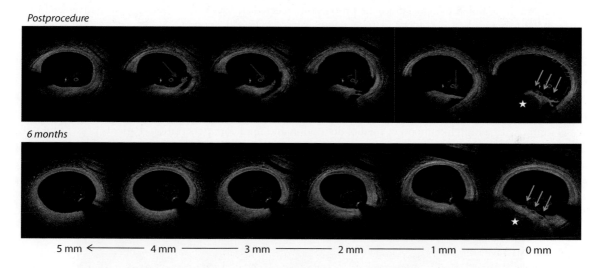

Figure 1.9 Serial examination of OCT-detected stent edge dissection. Top panel: Consecutive OCT cross section images of the 5 mm distal edge after implantation of a 3.0 × 18 mm polymeric bioresorbable scaffold to treat a proximal right coronary artery (RCA) lesion. Note the polymeric struts (green arrows) at the scaffold border landing over an eccentric calcified plaque (white star). Disruption of the arterial lumen surface is seen over a long (4.0 mm) segment at the distal scaffold edge. The dissection presented as a flap located in the region of compliance mismatch at the junction between the eccentric fibrocalcific plaque and the normal vessel, and it was restricted to the atheroma. Maximum flap opening measured 0.12 mm. This dissection was not visible by angiography. Bottom panel: Matched OCT cross sections after 6 months. Note the complete healing of the scaffold edge dissection, with a smooth lumen lining, and maintenance of the original lumen dimensions. In addition to the distance from the scaffold edge measurement, the pericardial structure at one o'clock can be used to coregister the OCT cross sections between the two time points.

1.4.3.2   In-stent dissections, tissue prolapse, and in-stent thrombus

Plaque fracture and dissection of the arterial wall are the key mechanisms of lumen enlargement during PCI. As a result, disruption of the endoluminal vessel wall continuity (in-stent dissection) and tissue prolapse between the stent struts are almost universally encountered after stenting, with incidences ranging from 44% to 98%[41,92,93,95] and 42% to 100%,[41,85–87,92,93,95] respectively. OCT findings suggestive of intra-stent thrombus are also frequent after successful stent implantation, ranging from 35% to 49%.[41,85,87,92,93,95] Figure 1.10 illustrates the OCT characteristics and definitions of such findings.

Several animal and pathological studies have associated the degree of vessel injury with ISR.[96,97] In addition, concerns have been raised that disruption of the vessel wall with loss of endothelial integrity, and lipid core penetration with prolapse of its contents between the stent struts, could lead to increased stent thrombogenicity.[98,99]

However, although associated with periprocedural MI,[41] most in-stent dissections heal over the midterm follow-up[93] and are not associated with adverse clinical events at 1 year.[93,95]

Tissue prolapse and in-stent thrombus are more frequent in ACSs and thrombus-containing lesions.[85] Importantly, additional balloon inflations may worsen the magnitude of tissue or thrombus prolapse by embedding the stent deeper into the underlying soft plaque, and increase the risk of distal embolization. In the study by Porto et al., the presence of in-stent thrombus after successful coronary stent implantation was independently associated with periprocedural MI (OR 5.5, 95% CI 1.2–24.9). Nonetheless, various small reports have failed to associate tissue protrusion detected by OCT after stenting with adverse clinical events.[85,87,92] In a more recent OCT registry of 1001 stents implanted in 900 lesions from 786 patients, Soeda et al. categorized in-stent tissue protrusions into three groups claiming to estimate different severities of vessel injury. Smooth protrusions were defined as bowing of plaque into the lumen between the stent struts without intimal disruption, and represented minimal vessel injury. Disrupted fibrous tissue protrusions (disruption of the underlying fibrous tissue protruding between the struts) represented mild vessel injury, and irregular protrusions (protrusion of material with an irregular surface between the struts) indicated moderate to severe vessel injury with a high likelihood of medial disruption and lipid core penetration. Patients presenting with acute MI had a higher incidence of irregular protrusions (67% vs. 46.7%, $p < 0.001$) and a smaller incidence of disrupted fibrous tissue protrusion (53% vs. 64.2%, $p = 0.007$) than patients presenting with stable angina. As expected, lesions with irregular protrusions had a higher incidence of thrombus than those without irregular

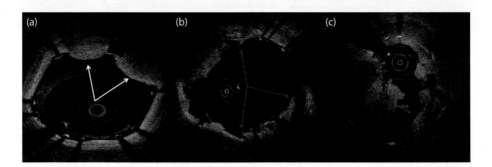

Figure 1.10 Other qualitative findings on poststenting OCT. Tissue prolapse (a) is characterized as projections of tissue into the lumen between the stent struts without disruption of the continuity of the luminal surface (white arrows). In-stent dissection (b) is defined by disruption of the endoluminal vessel wall continuity (red arrows) in the in-stent segment. In-stent thrombus (c) is characterized as irregular masses attached to the stent struts or floating into the lumen. It can present with dorsal shadowing, depending on the timing and content of red blood cells.

protrusions (78.1% vs. 38.1%, $p < 0.001$)—although the differentiation between irregular protrusion and thrombus may not be possible in cases where thrombus is attached to the luminal surface. In the multivariable logistic regression analysis, irregular protrusions were identified as independent predictors of device-oriented clinical endpoints (cardiac death, target vessel-related MI, target lesion revascularization, and stent thrombosis) (OR 2.64, 95% CI 1.40–5.01) and target lesion revascularization (OR 2.66, 95% CI 1.40–5.05). It is important to note that these results come from a retrospective analysis, and the proposed tissue protrusion classification has not been validated. Furthermore, the impact of tissue protrusion on the magnitude of lumen compromise was not presented. Whether the increased incidence of adverse events in patients with irregular protrusions is derived from mechanical obstruction of lumen flow or the baseline clinical risk of such patients cannot be determined.

1.5 POTENTIAL CLINICAL IMPACT OF OCT USE FOR PCI PLANNING AND GUIDANCE

The clear, detailed, and accurate information provided by OCT is easier to interpret, with a shorter learning curve, than other intravascular imaging modalities. As a consequence, an elevated rate of interaction of operators in response to the data provided by the OCT has been reported.

In the prospective series by Stefano et al.,[100] OCT was used pre-PCI, post-PCI, or both pre- and post-PCI in 150 consecutive patients enrolled during a 2-month period aiming to assess the safety, success, and impact of FD-OCT on patient management in the cardiac catheterization laboratory. Notably, operators changed the initial angiographic-based strategy in 81.8% of the cases after performing pre-PCI OCT. The most frequent changes were in the predicted stent length (48.5%) and diameter (27.3%). Most of the changes in stent length (30.3%) were for longer stent lengths, as is frequently the case with any invasive imaging modality, which allows visualization of more diseased segments than angiography. Of note, it is important to observe that pre-PCI OCT shortened the predicted stent length in 18.2% of the cases. When OCT was used poststenting, further interventions were performed in an additional 54.8% of the treated target vessels. Poststenting, malapposition was detected in 39.2% of the cases (89.4% of which underwent further balloon dilatation), and stent edge dissection in 32.5% (21.1% treated with additional stents).

In the largest and more recent ILUMIEN I study, OCT and documentary FFR were performed pre- and post-PCI in 418 patients. Based on pre-PCI OCT, the initial strategy was altered in 55% of patients (57% of all stenoses). Once again, longer stents were selected (43%), but a nonnegligible proportion of lesions had their predicted stent lengths shortened (25%). After clinically successful stent implantation, post-PCI OCT and FFR were repeated. Suboptimal results as per the operator's interpretation of OCT findings were frequent (14.5% malapposition, 7.6% underexpansion, and 2.7% edge dissection) and prompted further optimization in 25% of patients (27% of all stenoses), by either additional balloon dilatation (81%) or placement of additional stents (12%). Interestingly, the final FFR (~0.89) was not significantly different with respect to the timing of OCT use to plan or optimize the PCI. Of note, in the subset of cases with paired final FFR and OCT measurements following optimization, FFR values improved from 0.86 ± 0.07 to 0.90 ± 0.10 following correction of OCT findings that were deemed unsatisfactory by the operator.[101]

These reports reaffirm the importance of pre-PCI imaging for strategy planning, as demonstrated by the elevated change and refinement of the initially predicted strategy. Post-PCI OCT also offered additional opportunities for optimization of the PCI results. However, other than correcting small minimal in-stent lumen areas and regions of underexpansion (strong predictors of late stent failure), exaggerated stent malapposition, and extensive and deep edge dissections with lumen compromise, overreaction to other smaller abnormalities (although frequently detected by post-PCI OCT) may not be of clinical relevance.

Currently, there is a paucity of data on OCT predictors of stent failure, as well as prospectively validated protocols for stent sizing and optimization.

In the CLI-OPCI observational study, Prati et al.[102] compared the clinical outcomes of PCI guided by angiography alone with those of PCI guided by angiography plus OCT in a matched population of 670 patients (335 for each group). A pragmatic protocol was used at the involved centers to make practices uniform and enforce similar criteria for intervention when OCT use was considered to guide PCI. No quantitative criteria were proposed for stent sizing or positioning, which were left to the operator's discretion. The protocol recommended the following actions to specific OCT disclosed issues: (1) edge dissection (linear rim of tissue with a width of ≥200 μm and a clear separation from the vessel wall) and reference lumen narrowing (lumen area of <4.0 mm^2) required implantation of an additional stent; (2) stent underexpansion (MLA of ≤90% of the average reference lumen area or ≥100% of the lumen area of the smallest reference) required further dilatation with a noncompliant balloon the same diameter of the stent inflated ≥18 atm, or with a semicompliant balloon ≥0.25 mm larger than the stent inflated at ≥14 atm; (3) stent malapposition (strut-to-lumen distance of >200 μm) required further dilatation with a noncompliant or semicompliant balloon with a diameter ≥0.25 larger than that of the previously used balloon, at ≥14 atm; (4) thrombus required further dilatation with a noncompliant or semicompliant balloon of the same diameter as the stent at 8–16 atm for 60 seconds. Features disclosed by OCT, and not detected by angiography, represented edge dissections in 14.2%, lumen narrowing in 2.8%, stent malapposition in 29.7%, stent underexpansion in 11.4%, and intracoronary thrombus in 22.0%. These findings led to additional interventions in 34% of the cases (additional stents in 12.6% and additional balloon dilatations in 22.1%). At the end of 1 year, patients submitted to PCI with angiography plus OCT guidance experienced significantly lower rates of cardiac death (1.2% vs. 4.5%, $p = 0.01$), cardiac death or MI (6.6% vs. 13%, $p = 0.006$), and the composite of cardiac death, MI, and repeat revascularization (9.6% vs. 14.8%, $p = 0.044$). These favorable clinical outcomes persisted after extensive multivariable regression analysis (OR 0.49, 95% CI 0.25–0.96, $p = 0.037$), propensity score–adjusted analysis with bootstrap resampling (OR 0.37, 95% CI 0.10–0.90, $p = 0.050$), and Cox proportional hazards analysis (hazard ratio [HR] 0.51, 95% CI 0.28–0.93, $p = 0.028$).

The currently ongoing DOCTORS study is a prospective, randomized, multicenter, open-label clinical trial that evaluates the utility of OCT to optimize results of angioplasty of a lesion responsible for a non-ST-elevation ACS. Patients ($n = 250$) are randomized to OCT-guided PCI or angiography-guided PCI. A protocol for stent sizing and deployment is not enforced, but guidelines for procedural optimization are applied as follows: (1) additional balloon inflations should be performed in the case of stent underexpansion, defined as a minimal stent area of ≤80% of the reference lumen area; (2) additional stent implantation should be performed to rectify incomplete lesion coverage (including edge dissection); (3) use of glycoprotein IIb/IIIa inhibitors and/or thromboaspiration should be systematically considered in the case of thrombus presence; and (4) rotational atherectomy should be considered in the case of circumferential calcification. The primary endpoint is the functional result of PCI as assessed by FFR measured at the end of the procedure.[103]

Although prospective, randomized, adequately powered clinical trials for the assessment of the impact of OCT-guided PCI on clinical outcomes is still needed, the ongoing large prospective OCT registry led by Dr. I. K. Jang, which enrolled around 3000 patients, will start to shine some light on the clinical impact of OCT.

REFERENCES

1. Stefanini GG, Holmes DR Jr. Drug-eluting coronary-artery stents. *New England Journal of Medicine* 2013;368:254–65.
2. Colombo A et al. Intracoronary stenting without anticoagulation accomplished with intravascular ultrasound guidance. *Circulation* 1995;91:1676–88.
3. Zhang Y et al. Comparison of intravascular ultrasound versus angiography-guided drug-eluting stent implantation: A meta-analysis of one randomised trial and ten observational studies involving 19,619 patients. *EuroIntervention* 2012;8:855–65.
4. Klersy C et al. Use of IVUS guided coronary stenting with drug eluting stent: A systematic review and meta-analysis of randomized controlled clinical trials and high quality observational studies. *International Journal of Cardiology* 2013;170:54–63.
5. Jang JS et al. Intravascular ultrasound-guided implantation of drug-eluting stents to improve outcome: A meta-analysis. *JACC Cardiovascular Interventions* 2014;7:233–43.
6. Ahn JM et al. Meta-analysis of outcomes after intravascular ultrasound-guided versus angiography-guided drug-eluting stent implantation in 26,503 patients enrolled in three randomized trials and 14 observational studies. *American Journal of Cardiology* 2014;113:1338–47.
7. Dattilo PB et al. Contemporary patterns of fractional flow reserve and intravascular ultrasound use among patients undergoing percutaneous coronary intervention in the United States: Insights from the National Cardiovascular Data Registry. *Journal of the American College of Cardiology* 2012;60:2337–9.
8. Tearney GJ et al. Consensus standards for acquisition, measurement, and reporting of intravascular optical coherence tomography studies: A report from the International Working Group for Intravascular Optical Coherence Tomography Standardization and Validation. *Journal of the American College of Cardiology* 2012;59:1058–72.
9. Yamaguchi T et al. Safety and feasibility of an intravascular optical coherence tomography image wire system in the clinical setting. *American Journal of Cardiology* 2008;101:562–7.
10. Capodanno D et al. Comparison of optical coherence tomography and intravascular ultrasound for the assessment of in-stent tissue coverage after stent implantation. *EuroIntervention* 2009;5:538–43.
11. Gonzalo N et al. Quantitative ex vivo and in vivo comparison of lumen dimensions measured by optical coherence tomography and intravascular ultrasound in human coronary arteries. *Revista Espanola de Cardiologia* 2009;62:615–24.
12. Farooq V et al. 3D reconstructions of optical frequency domain imaging to improve understanding of conventional PCI. *JACC Cardiovascular Imaging* 2011;4:1044–6.
13. Bezerra HG et al. Optical coherence tomography versus intravascular ultrasound to evaluate coronary artery disease and percutaneous coronary intervention. *JACC Cardiovascular Interventions* 2013;6:228–36.
14. Kubo T et al. OCT compared with IVUS in a coronary lesion assessment: The OPUS-CLASS study. *JACC Cardiovascular Imaging* 2013;6:1095–104.
15. Tsuchida K et al. In vivo validation of a novel three-dimensional quantitative coronary angiography system (CardiOp-B): Comparison with a conventional two-dimensional system (CAAS II) and with special reference to optical coherence tomography. *EuroIntervention* 2007;3:100–8.
16. Sawada T et al. Factors that influence measurements and accurate evaluation of stent apposition by optical coherence tomography. Assessment using a phantom model. *Circulation Journal* 2009;73:1841–7.
17. Tahara S et al. In vitro validation of new Fourier-domain optical coherence tomography. *EuroIntervention* 2011;6:875–82.
18. Gonzalo N et al. Morphometric assessment of coronary stenosis relevance with optical coherence tomography: A comparison with fractional flow reserve and intravascular ultrasound. *Journal of the American College of Cardiology* 2012;59:1080–9.
19. Shiono Y et al. Optical coherence tomography-derived anatomical criteria for functionally significant coronary stenosis assessed by fractional flow reserve. *Circulation Journal* 2012;76:2218–25.
20. Reith S et al. Relationship between optical coherence tomography derived intraluminal and intramural criteria and haemodynamic relevance as determined by fractional flow reserve in intermediate coronary stenoses of patients with type 2 diabetes. *Heart* 2013;99:700–7.
21. Pawlowski T et al. Optical coherence tomography criteria for defining functional severity of intermediate lesions: A comparative study with FFR *The International Journal of Cardiovascular Imaging* 2013;29:1685–91.
22. Pyxaras SA et al. Quantitative angiography and optical coherence tomography for the functional assessment of nonobstructive coronary stenoses: Comparison with fractional flow reserve. *American Heart Journal* 2013;166:1010–8 e1011.

23. Reith S et al. Correlation between optical coherence tomography-derived intraluminal parameters and fractional flow reserve measurements in intermediate grade coronary lesions: A comparison between diabetic and non-diabetic patients. *Clinical Research in Cardiology: Official Journal of the German Cardiac Society* 2015;104:59–70.

24. Jang IK et al. Visualization of coronary atherosclerotic plaques in patients using optical coherence tomography: Comparison with intravascular ultrasound. *Journal of the American College of Cardiology* 2002;39:604–9.

25. Yabushita H et al. Characterization of human atherosclerosis by optical coherence tomography. *Circulation* 2002;106:1640–5.

26. Kume T et al. Assessment of coronary intima-media thickness by optical coherence tomography: Comparison with intravascular ultrasound. *Circulation Journal* 2005;69:903–7.

27. Cilingiroglu M et al. Detection of vulnerable plaque in a murine model of atherosclerosis with optical coherence tomography. *Catheterization and Cardiovascular Interventions* 2006;67:915–23.

28. Kume T et al. Measurement of the thickness of the fibrous cap by optical coherence tomography. *American Heart Journal* 2006;152:755.e1–4.

29. Tearney GJ et al. Quantification of macrophage content in atherosclerotic plaques by optical coherence tomography. *Circulation* 2002;107:113–9.

30. MacNeill BD et al. Focal and multi-focal plaque macrophage distributions in patients with acute and stable presentations of coronary artery disease. *Journal of the American College of Cardiology* 2004;44:972–9.

31. Kubo T et al. Assessment of culprit lesion morphology in acute myocardial infarction: Ability of optical coherence tomography compared with intravascular ultrasound and coronary angioscopy. *Journal of the American College of Cardiology* 2007;50:933–9.

32. Kume T et al. Assessment of coronary arterial thrombus by optical coherence tomography. *American Journal of Cardiology* 2006;97:1713–7.

33. Jang IK et al. In vivo characterization of coronary atherosclerotic plaque by use of optical coherence tomography. *Circulation* 2005;111:1551–5.

34. Ino Y et al. Difference of culprit lesion morphologies between ST-segment elevation myocardial infarction and non-ST-segment elevation acute coronary syndrome: An optical coherence tomography study. *JACC Cardiovascular Interventions* 2011;4:76–82.

35. Tanaka A et al. Morphology of exertion-triggered plaque rupture in patients with acute coronary syndrome: An optical coherence tomography study. *Circulation* 2008;118:2368–73.

36. Niccoli G et al. Plaque rupture and intact fibrous cap assessed by optical coherence tomography portend different outcomes in patients with acute coronary syndrome. *European Heart Journal* 2015;36:1377–84.

37. Mehanna E et al. Volumetric characterization of human coronary calcification by frequency-domain optical coherence tomography. *Circulation Journal* 2013;77:2334–40.

38. Mintz GS. Intravascular imaging of coronary calcification and its clinical implications. *JACC Cardiovascular Imaging* 2015;8:461–71.

39. Tanaka A et al. Lipid-rich plaque and myocardial perfusion after successful stenting in patients with non-ST-segment elevation acute coronary syndrome: An optical coherence tomography study. *European Heart Journal* 2009;30:1348–55.

40. Ozaki Y et al. Thin-cap fibroatheroma as high-risk plaque for microvascular obstruction in patients with acute coronary syndrome. *Circulation Cardiovascular Imaging* 2011;4:620–7.

41. Porto I et al. Predictors of periprocedural (type IVa) myocardial infarction, as assessed by frequency-domain optical coherence tomography. *Circulation Cardiovascular Interventions* 2012;5:89–96, S1–6.

42. Lee T et al. Impact of coronary plaque morphology assessed by optical coherence tomography on cardiac troponin elevation in patients with elective stent implantation. *Circulation Cardiovascular Interventions* 2011;4:378–86.

43. Chamie D et al. Incidence, predictors, morphological characteristics, and clinical outcomes of stent edge dissections detected by optical coherence tomography. *JACC Cardiovascular Interventions* 2013;6:800–13.

44. van Ditzhuijzen NS et al. The impact of Fourier-domain optical coherence tomography catheter induced motion artefacts on quantitative measurements of a PLLA-based bioresorbable scaffold. *International Journal of Cardiovascular Imaging* 2014;30:1013–26.

45. Mintz GS et al. Atherosclerosis in angiographically "normal" coronary artery reference segments: An intravascular ultrasound study with clinical correlations. *Journal of the American College of Cardiology* 1995;25:1479–85.

46. Habara M et al. Impact of frequency-domain optical coherence tomography guidance for optimal coronary stent implantation in comparison with intravascular ultrasound guidance. *Circulation Cardiovascular Interventions* 2012;5:193–201.

47. Maehara A et al. Comparison of stent expansion guided by optical coherence tomography versus intravascular ultrasound: The ILUMIEN II Study (Observational Study of Optical Coherence Tomography [OCT] in Patients Undergoing Fractional Flow Reserve [FFR] and Percutaneous Coronary Intervention). *JACC Cardiovascular Interventions* 2015;8:1704–14.

48. Ali ZA et al. Optical coherence tomography compared with intravascular ultrasound and with angiography to guide coronary stent implantation (ilumien iii: Optimize pci): A randomised controlled trial. *Lancet* 2016;388:2618–28.

49. Kasaoka S et al. Angiographic and intravascular ultrasound predictors of in-stent restenosis. *Journal of the American College of Cardiology* 1998;32:1630–5.

50. de Feyter PJ et al. Reference chart derived from post-stent-implantation intravascular ultrasound predictors of 6-month expected restenosis on quantitative coronary angiography. *Circulation* 1999;100:1777–83.

51. Castagna MT et al. The contribution of "mechanical" problems to in-stent restenosis: An intravascular ultrasonographic analysis of 1090 consecutive in-stent restenosis lesions. *American Heart Journal* 2001;142:970–4.

52. Morino Y et al. An optimal diagnostic threshold for minimal stent area to predict target lesion revascularization following stent implantation in native coronary lesions. *American Journal of Cardiology* 2001;88:301–3.

53. Ziada KM et al. Prognostic value of absolute versus relative measures of the procedural result after successful coronary stenting: Importance of vessel size in predicting long-term freedom from target vessel revascularization. *American Heart Journal* 2001;141:823–31.

54. Cheneau E et al. Predictors of subacute stent thrombosis: Results of a systematic intravascular ultrasound study. *Circulation* 2003;108:43–7.

55. Fujii K et al. Contribution of stent underexpansion to recurrence after sirolimus-eluting stent implantation for in-stent restenosis. *Circulation* 2004;109:1085–8.

56. Sonoda S et al. Impact of final stent dimensions on long-term results following sirolimus-eluting stent implantation: Serial intravascular ultrasound analysis from the sirius trial. *Journal of the American College of Cardiology* 2004;43:1959–63.

57. Fujii K et al. Stent underexpansion and residual reference segment stenosis are related to stent thrombosis after sirolimus-eluting stent implantation: An intravascular ultrasound study. *Journal of the American College of Cardiology* 2005;45:995–8.

58. Hong MK et al. Intravascular ultrasound predictors of angiographic restenosis after sirolimus-eluting stent implantation. *European Heart Journal* 2006;27:1305–10.

59. Okabe T et al. Intravascular ultrasound parameters associated with stent thrombosis after drug-eluting stent deployment. *American Journal of Cardiology* 2007;100:615–20.

60. Doi H et al. Impact of post-intervention minimal stent area on 9-month follow-up patency of paclitaxel-eluting stents: An integrated intravascular ultrasound analysis from the TAXUS IV, V, and VI and TAXUS ATLAS workhorse, long lesion, and direct stent trials. *JACC Cardiovascular Interventions* 2009;2:1269–75.

61. Liu X et al. A volumetric intravascular ultrasound comparison of early drug-eluting stent thrombosis versus restenosis. *JACC Cardiovascular Interventions* 2009;2:428–34.

62. Choi SY et al. Intravascular ultrasound findings of early stent thrombosis after primary percutaneous intervention in acute myocardial infarction: A Harmonizing Outcomes with Revascularization and Stents in Acute Myocardial Infarction (HORIZONS-AMI) substudy. *Circulation Cardiovascular Interventions* 2011;4:239–47.

63. Kang SJ et al. Comprehensive intravascular ultrasound assessment of stent area and its impact on restenosis and adverse cardiac events in 403 patients with unprotected left main disease. *Circulation Cardiovascular Interventions* 2011;4:562–9.

64. Choi SY et al. Usefulness of minimum stent cross sectional area as a predictor of angiographic restenosis after primary percutaneous coronary intervention in acute myocardial infarction (from the HORIZONS-AMI Trial IVUS substudy). *American Journal of Cardiology* 2012;109:455–60.

65. Kang SJ et al. Usefulness of minimal luminal coronary area determined by intravascular ultrasound to predict functional significance in stable and unstable angina pectoris. *American Journal of Cardiology* 2012;109:947–53.

66. Song HG et al. Intravascular ultrasound assessment of optimal stent area to prevent in-stent restenosis after zotarolimus-, everolimus-, and sirolimus-eluting stent implantation. *Catheterization and Cardiovascular Interventions* 2014;83:873–8.

67. Hong MK et al. Incidence, mechanism, predictors, and long-term prognosis of late stent malapposition after bare-metal stent implantation. *Circulation* 2004;109:881–6.

68. Mintz GS et al. Regional remodeling as the cause of late stent malapposition. *Circulation* 2003;107:2660–3.

69. Shah VM et al. Background incidence of late malapposition after bare-metal stent implantation. *Circulation* 2002;106:1753–5.

70. Kang SJ et al. Late and very late drug-eluting stent malapposition: Serial 2-year quantitative IVUS analysis. *Circulation Cardiovascular Interventions* 2010;3:335–40.

71. Ako J et al. Late incomplete stent apposition after sirolimus-eluting stent implantation: A serial intravascular ultrasound analysis. *Journal of the American College of Cardiology* 2005;46:1002–5.

72. Tanabe K et al. Incomplete stent apposition after implantation of paclitaxel-eluting stents or bare metal stents: Insights from the randomized TAXUS II trial. *Circulation* 2005;111:900–5.

73. Hong MK et al. Late stent malapposition after drug-eluting stent implantation: An intravascular ultrasound analysis with long-term follow-up. *Circulation* 2006;113:414–9.

74. Siqueira DA et al. Late incomplete apposition after drug-eluting stent implantation: Incidence and potential for adverse clinical outcomes. *European Heart Journal* 2007;28:1304–9.

75. Ozaki Y et al. The fate of incomplete stent apposition with drug-eluting stents: An optical coherence tomography-based natural history study. *European Heart Journal* 2010;31:1470–6.

76. Hassan AK et al. Late stent malapposition risk is higher after drug-eluting stent compared with bare-metal stent implantation and associates with late stent thrombosis. *European Heart Journal* 2010;31:1172–80.

77. Steinberg DH et al. Long-term impact of routinely detected early and late incomplete stent apposition: An integrated intravascular ultrasound analysis of the TAXUS IV, V, and VI and TAXUS ATLAS workhorse, long lesion, and direct stent studies. *JACC Cardiovascular Interventions* 2010;3:486–94.

78. Cook S et al. Impact of incomplete stent apposition on long-term clinical outcome after drug-eluting stent implantation. *European Heart Journal* 2012;33:1334–43.

79. Im E et al. Incidences, predictors, and clinical outcomes of acute and late stent malapposition detected by optical coherence tomography after drug-eluting stent implantation. *Circulation Cardiovascular Interventions* 2014;7:88–96.

80. Guagliumi G et al. Examination of the in vivo mechanisms of late drug-eluting stent thrombosis: Findings from optical coherence tomography and intravascular ultrasound imaging. *JACC Cardiovascular Interventions* 2012;5:12–20.

81. Cook S et al. Incomplete stent apposition and very late stent thrombosis after drug-eluting stent implantation. *Circulation* 2007;115:2426–34.

82. Alfonso F et al. Coronary aneurysms after drug-eluting stent implantation: Clinical, angiographic, and intravascular ultrasound findings. *Journal of the American College of Cardiology* 2009;53:2053–60.

83. Kimura M et al. Outcome after acute incomplete sirolimus-eluting stent apposition as assessed by serial intravascular ultrasound. *American Journal of Cardiology* 2006;98:436–42.

84. Guo N et al. Incidence, mechanisms, predictors, and clinical impact of acute and late stent malapposition after primary intervention in patients with acute myocardial infarction: An intravascular ultrasound substudy of the Harmonizing Outcomes with Revascularization and Stents in Acute Myocardial Infarction (HORIZONS-AMI) trial. *Circulation* 2010;122:1077–84.

85. Kubo T et al. Comparison of vascular response after sirolimus-eluting stent implantation between patients with unstable and stable angina pectoris: A serial optical coherence tomography study. *JACC Cardiovascular Imaging* 2008;1:475–84.

86. Kume T et al. Natural history of stent edge dissection, tissue protrusion and incomplete stent apposition detectable only on optical coherence tomography after stent implantation. *Circulation Journal* 2012;76:698–703.

87. Kawamori H et al. Natural consequence of post-intervention stent malapposition, thrombus, tissue prolapse, and dissection assessed by optical coherence tomography at mid-term follow-up. *European Heart Journal Cardiovascular Imaging* 2013;14:865–75.

88. Guagliumi G et al. Serial assessment of coronary artery response to paclitaxel-eluting stents using optical coherence tomography. *Circulation Cardiovascular Interventions* 2012;5:30–8.

89. Gutierrez-Chico JL et al. Vascular tissue reaction to acute malapposition in human coronary arteries: Sequential assessment with optical coherence tomography. *Circulation Cardiovascular Interventions* 2012;5:20–9, S1–8.

90. Inoue T et al. Impact of strut-vessel distance and underlying plaque type on the resolution of acute strut malapposition: Serial optimal coherence tomography analysis after everolimus-eluting stent implantation. *International Journal of Cardiovascular Imaging* 2014;30:857–65.

91. Foin N et al. Incomplete stent apposition causes high shear flow disturbances and delay in neointimal coverage as a function of strut to wall detachment distance: Implications for the management of incomplete stent apposition. *Circulation. Cardiovascular Interventions*. 2014;7:180–9.

92. Gonzalo N et al. Optical coherence tomography assessment of the acute effects of stent implantation on the vessel wall: A systematic quantitative approach. *Heart* 2009;95:1913–9.

93. De Cock D et al. Healing course of acute vessel wall injury after drug-eluting stent implantation assessed by optical coherence tomography. *European Heart Journal Cardiovascular Imaging* 2014;15:800–9.

94. Radu MD et al. Natural history of optical coherence tomography-detected non-flow-limiting edge dissections following drug-eluting stent implantation. *EuroIntervention* 2014;9:1085–94.

95. Soeda T et al. Incidence and clinical significance of poststent optical coherence tomography findings: One-year follow-up study from a multicenter registry. *Circulation* 2015;132:1020–9.

96. Farb A et al. Pathology of acute and chronic coronary stenting in humans. *Circulation* 1999;99:44–52.

97. Schwartz RS et al. Restenosis and the proportional neointimal response to coronary artery injury: Results in a porcine model. *Journal of the American College of Cardiology* 1992;19:267–74.

98. Farb A et al. Pathological mechanisms of fatal late coronary stent thrombosis in humans. *Circulation* 2003;108:1701–6.

99. Nakano M et al. Causes of early stent thrombosis in patients presenting with acute coronary syndrome: An ex vivo human autopsy study. *Journal of the American College of Cardiology* 2014;63:2510–20.

100. Stefano GT et al. Unrestricted utilization of frequency domain optical coherence tomography in coronary interventions. *International Journal of Cardiovascular Imaging* 2013;29:741–52.

101. Wijns W et al. Optical coherence tomography imaging during percutaneous coronary intervention impacts physician decision-making: ILUMIEN I study. *European Heart Journal* 2015;36:3346–55.

102. Prati F et al. Angiography alone versus angiography plus optical coherence tomography to guide decision-making during percutaneous coronary intervention: The Centro per la Lotta contro l'Infarto-Optimisation of Percutaneous Coronary Intervention (CLI-OPCI) study. *EuroIntervention* 2012;8:823–9.

103. Meneveau N et al. Does optical coherence tomography optimize results of stenting? Rationale and study design. *American Heart Journal* 2014;168:175–81.e1–2.

Chapter 2

OCT imaging for assessment of plaque modification

Ruben Ramos and Lino Patrício

2.1 INTRODUCTION

The aim of this section is to illustrate the ability of optical coherence tomography (OCT) in the identification of typical vascular responses to coronary interventions. In particular, we focus on how this high-definition imaging tool can help the operator guide the intervention and assist in real-time clinical decisions.

2.2 PLAIN ORDINARY BALLOON AND DRUG-ELUTING BALLOON ANGIOPLASTY

Current percutaneous coronary interventions (PCIs) are largely based on stent implantation. However, balloon angioplasty lingers as a pre- and poststent adjunctive strategy or sometimes as a valuable stand-alone alternative to stenting. Balloon angioplasty is frequently associated with plaque fracture and intimal surface disruption (Figure 2.1a). Intracoronary imaging may be a valuable ancillary instrument for balloon-based intervention in the detection of postintervention abnormalities that may go underrecognized by angiography alone (Figure 2.2) or in the fine-tuning of stent-based procedural optimization (Figure 2.1b). Intravascular ultrasound (IVUS) has traditionally been used for the diagnosis of coronary dissections when angiography is dubious. However, the 10 times superior axial resolution of OCT compared with IVUS may lead to more frequent recognition of unintended vascular injury during PCI. The clinical implications of these improved capabilities of OCT to detect vessel injury, especially if not angiographically evident, are not completely established.

Drug-eluting balloons (DEBs) may have an important role in small vessel angioplasty, in-stent restenosis (Figure 2.3), and ostial-bifurcational lesions (Figure 2.4). Intravascular imaging may be especially important in nonstent interventions since balloon sizing and resultant acute luminal gain may determine short- and long-term success. Even after an optimal angiographic result, intracoronary imaging may lead to modification in treatment strategies in up to 73% of target lesions (Figures 2.1 and 2.2).[1] It has been suggested that morphological patterns of in-stent restenosis as defined by OCT can predict the response to DEB (Figure 2.3).[2]

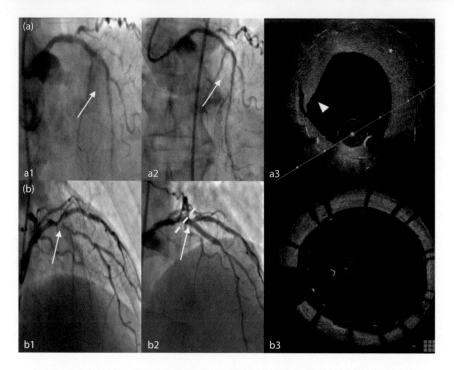

Figure 2.1 Illustrative cases of acceptable final angiography after PCI with suboptimal results as assessed by OCT.
(a) Nondiabetic patient presenting with non-ST-elevation myocardial infarction (NSTEMI) initially treated with an under-sized 2.5 mm bare-metal stent (BMS) for an isolated mid–left anterior descendent artery (LAD) stenosis. Nine months later, ischemia-driven angiography detected significant in-stent restenosis (ISR), which was treated with a 2.75 mm DES. Recurrent angina prompted a third coronary angiography with diagnosis of recurrent ISR (arrow in a1). Note the double stent layer in a3. It was decided to treat the lesion with a 3 mm DEB after predilatation with a 3 mm NC balloon. A good final angiographic result was noted (arrow in a2). Control OCT, however, showed significant residual and eccentric (*) neointimal fibrotic plaque with an associated intrastent dissection flap (arrowhead in a3). (b) Severe LAD stenosis just distal to bifurcation with the first diagonal branch (arrow in b1). Good angiographic result after 3 × 23 mm DES implantation, with distal stent–artery mismatch suggesting good stent sizing (b2). OCT revealed unsuspected significant stent malapposition pertaining to nearly five-sixths of the lumen circumference at the proximal stent edge (b3).

2.2.1   Cutting balloon or scoring balloon angioplasty

A cutting balloon (CB) is a noncompliant (NC) balloon with longitudinally bonded microtomes on the outer balloon surface, and it is designed to score atherosclerotic plaque, render plaque extension easier, reduce elastic recoil, minimize intimal injury, prevent progressive dissections, and facilitate stent delivery and expansion (Figure 2.5).[3] In-stent restenosis (Figures 2.3 and 2.4) and ostial bifurcational lesions (especially if Medina 0,0,1) still represent challenging subsets of lesions even in the era of drug-eluting stents (DESs). CB may have a role in these settings. Lesion preparation with CB, followed by optimal dilatation with an NC balloon (balloon–artery ratio 1:1) and subsequent DEB delivery, is often a strategy that reduces the risk of complex stenting procedures in bifurcations or avoids repeated stent overlapping in cases of in-stent restenosis (Figure 2.6).[4]

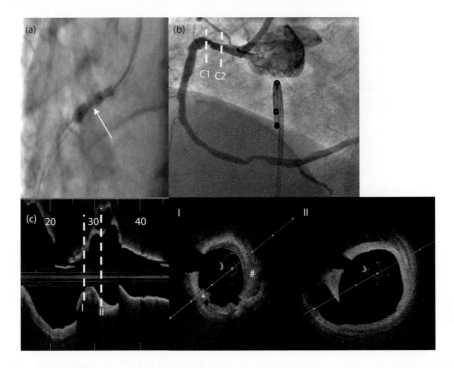

Figure 2.2 Balloon-induced coronary dissection unmasked by OCT. (a) Patient presenting with inferior ST-elevation myocardial infarction (STEMI) and an occluded proximal right coronary artery (RCA). Thrombolysis in myocardial infarction (TIMI) 3 flow was promptly achieved after crossing the lesion with a 0.014 in. wire. A severely stenostic lesion was noted and proved to be resistant to high-pressure balloon dilatation (arrow pointing to midballoon notch). (b) Angiographic result after balloon dilatation. Note that no coronary dissection is apparent. (c) Intracoronary imaging with OCT was then performed for further plaque characterization. Dashed lines C1 and C2 in the OCT longitudinal view represent the correspondent axial views. (C1) Note the residual luminal thrombus (*) and a severely fibrotic and calcified focal stenosis in the proximal right coronary artery (RCA) (#). (C2) Significant intimal dissection proximal to the stenosis unsuspected from the angiography. Before OCT imaging, the operator had the intention to proceed with RA to optimize lesion pretreatment before stent implantation. However, due to the OCT findings of a large intimal flap and residual intraluminal thrombi (*), rotablation was postponed to allow for adequate sealing of the intimal flap and thrombus resolution.

2.2.2   Rotational atherectomy

Severely calcified lesions are an important technical challenge to the interventionalist (Figures 2.2, 2.3, and 2.7). First, fibrocalcific plaques can lead to incomplete dilatation of the stenotic lesion, resulting in smaller acute luminal gains and increasing the risk of restenosis (Figure 2.4; also see Figure 2.19a).[5] Second, inappropriate stent expansion can lead to stent thrombosis.[6,7] Third, resistant lesions may require high-pressure balloon inflations, thereby greatly increasing the risk of vessel injury and rupture (Figure 2.2; also see Figure 2.19h). Rotational atherectomy (RA) is well suited for treating these types of lesions by preparing the vessel bed for optimal stent deployment. RA improves arterial compliance, allowing the transluminal passage of equipment and more uniform and symmetric stent deployment.[8]

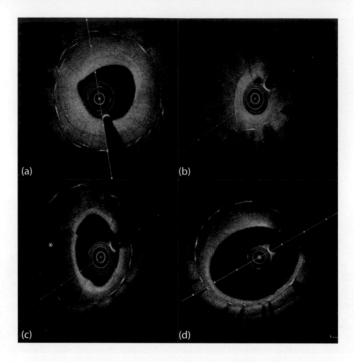

Figure 2.3 Morphological patterns of neointimal restenotic tissue as defined by OCT. (a) Homogenous neointimal tissue—uniform optical properties and no focal variations in backscattering pattern. (b and c) Layered restenotic pattern—concentric layers with different optical properties: an adluminal high-scattering layer and an abluminal low-scattering layer. Note in (c) the predominantly lipid content in the outer layer (*). (d) Heterogenous tissue—focally changing optical properties with multiple backscattering intensities. It has been suggested that nonhomogenous patterns of in-stent restenosis may be less responsive to treatment with paclitaxel-eluting balloon than lesions with a homogenous structure.[2]

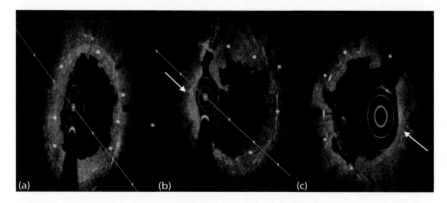

Figure 2.4 In-stent restenosis lesions after treatment with CB. (a) Concentric lesion. Note the multiple uniform cutting-induced craters along the luminal contour resultant from successive CB dilatations (*). (b and c) Eccentric lesions with non-uniform cutting effect. Most of the cutting effect is localized in just one side of the vessel wall (*), sparing the opposite side (arrows). Note also an associated intimal dissection flap in (b).

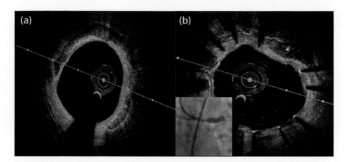

Figure 2.5 Severely calcified stenosis resulting in stent underexpansion. Patient with intermediate stenosis in the body of the left main coronary artery. Preintervention OCT was performed for stent sizing. (a) Note the subintimal calcified plaque involving approximately three-fourths of the vessel circumference. Despite this finding and possibly due to moderate severity of the stenosis and underecognition of calcification severity by angiography, the operator decided to proceed with direct stenting. (b) Stent underexpansion by angiography and OCT. Note the calcified plaque (*) preventing the full stent expansion. This persisted despite high-pressure postdilatation with a 4.0 mm NC balloon (inbox). It is possible that this suboptimal result could have been avoided by lesion preparation with CB or RA.

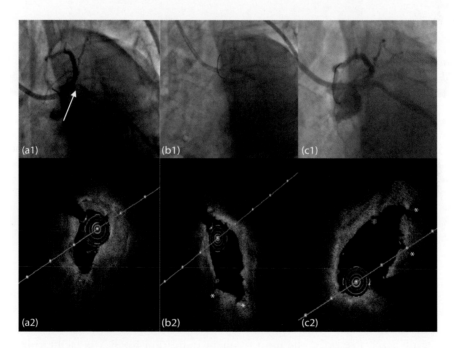

Figure 2.6 OCT-guided cutting-DEB approach for ostial circumflex artery lesion (Medina 0,0,1). Male patient, 76 years old, nondiabetic, presenting with stable angina. A single-photon emission computed tomography (SPECT) study showed evidence of inferolateral ischemia. (a) Significant calcified lesion (arrow) in ostial circumflex artery. Stenting of left circumflex artery (LCX) ostium was avoided due to possible compromise of proximal left anterior descendent artery (LAD). (b) Lesion preparation with a 2.5 mm CB to minimize acute elastic recoil. Note the eccentricity of the vessel and the intimal craters induced by the CB localized only to one pole of the vessel circumference (* in b2). (c1) Final angiographic result after postdilatation with a 3 mm NC balloon to maximize acute luminal area gain and subsequent delivery of a 3 mm DEB to reduce neointimal proliferation and late luminal loss. The LAD ostium remained unaffected. (c2) Final result by OCT. The minimal luminal area was 7.4 mm², and there was no evidence of intimal dissection to justify bailout stent implantation.

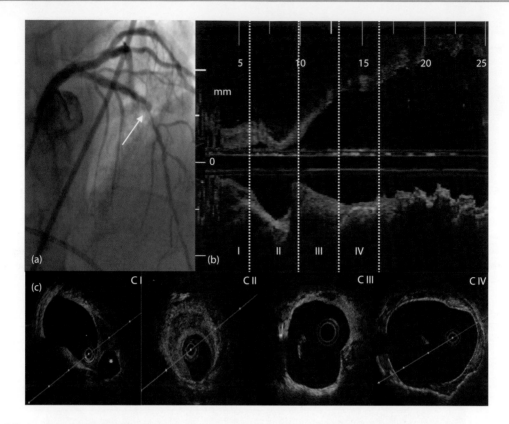

Figure 2.7 Angiographic and OCT findings of a severely calcified lesion in a vessel with diffusely atherosclerotic disease.
(a) The angiogram shows a calcified stenosis located in an angulated segment in the midportion of the left anterior descendent artery (LAD) that could not be crossed by a 2.0 mm balloon (A, white arrow). (b) Longitudinal OCT view of the evaluated segment. The numbered dashed lines identify the specific location of the cross-sectional images represented in (c). (CI) Calcified plaque involving a segment immediately distal to the critical stenosis. Note that the calcification involves the carina, but the ostium of the diagonal branch is relatively spared (*). (CII) Site of critical stenosis. The fibrotic and calcified plaque is well delineated. The signal-poor regions with sharp borders can be very well visualized by OCT and correspond to the calcific component part. (CIII) Superficial calcified plaque protruding to the lumen at four o'clock. (CIV) Nonstenotic segment proximal to the stenosis. This is a concentric and superficial plaque surrounding the entire lumen circumference.

The arterial response to RA is nonuniform and depends on several factors, including burr rotational speed, burr-to-artery ratio (Figures 2.8 and 2.9), lesion angulation and eccentricity (Figure 2.10), bifurcation involvement (Figures 2.8 and 2.10), stenosis severity (Figure 2.11), and plaque composition and distribution (Figure 2.12). Presently, the most frequent indication for RA is facilitating stent delivery and expansion in fibrocalcified lesions. This can be achieved by plaque debulking (Figures 2.9 and 2.13) or simply by plaque modification without major debulking (Figures 2.10, 2.11, and 2.14). Given the currently favored approach of the low burr-to-artery ratio strategy, the latter may be the main mechanism of action of RA.

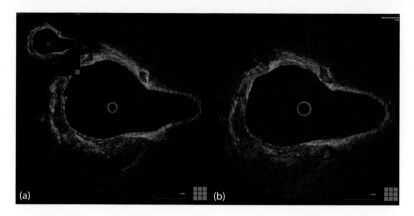

Figure 2.8 Lack of debulking effect within a bifurcational lesion. The burr-to-artery ratio of 0.625. (a) The pre-RA lumen area was 4.88 mm^2, and the calcification area was 3.88 mm^2. The inbox image shows that the 1.5 mm burr (represented by the purple circumference) does not intersect the vessel wall in the represented segment. (b) The post-RA lumen area was 4.88 mm^2, and the calcification area was 3.82 mm^2, similar to the pre-RA dimensions.

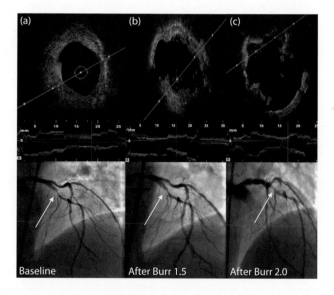

Figure 2.9 Effect of the burr-to-artery ratio on plaque debulking. (a) Fifty-five-year-old male patient presenting with acute coronary syndrome. The baseline angiogram revealed focal severe stenosis of the middle left anterior descendent artery (LAD) not crossable by a low-profile balloon (white arrow). The OCT image shows a predominantly fibrotic concentric lesion. (b) After RA with a 1.5 mm burr. Note the disrupted intimal surface and an acute luminal area gain, as seen in OCT and angiography. (c) In the OCT image, after RA one can note the debulking promoted by the 2.0 mm burr with an increase in minimal luminal area, major intimal disruption, and channel formation (*).

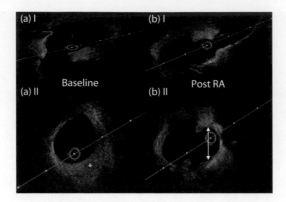

Figure 2.10 Different rotablation effect in two segments of the same lesion. (a) Baseline OCT. There is a concentric fibro-calcified plaque involving a bifurcation. The ostium of the collateral branch is relatively spared (I). In the same lesion, just immediately distal to the bifurcation and in the point of the minimal lumen area (II), the concentric plaque is mostly composed of dense fibrotic tissue (three to seven o'clock) with deep calcium nodules (*). (b) After rotablation. Note that in the bifurcation site the wire is pushed toward the wall of the side branch. There is no debulking, and minor plaque shifting toward the ostium of the side branch (I). In the most stenotic segment (II), however, there is considerable debulking of the fibrotic tissue and also channel formation. The diameter of the channel is approximately the same as that of the utilized burr (1.25 mm) (double arrow).

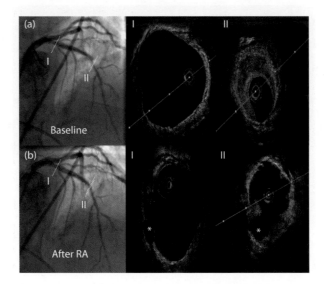

Figure 2.11 Different rotablation effect in two lesions of the same vessel. (a) Eighty-three-year-old male patient presenting with stable angina and single vessel disease. There is a diffusely diseased distal left anterior descendent artery (LAD), intermediate stenosis in the proximal segment (I), and critical stenosis in the middle segment (II). In the OCT images, one can note a nonobstructive lumen with an eccentric and superficial calcium plaque in the proximal lesion (level I in a) and a severe stenosis caused by a concentric fibrocalcified plaque (level II) in the midsegment. Given the OCT-confirmed finding of critical stenosis in a diffusely calcified mid-LAD segment, it was decided to proceed with RA as a first intention using a 1.25 mm burr to allow for optimal lesion preparation. (b) After RA. In the nonsevere proximal lesion, one can note a channel formation (*) with no significant debulking and minimal intimal disruption (level I in b). In the mid-LAD lesion, there is channel formation (*), but there is also associated significant debulking of the fibrocalcified plaque with evident extensive intimal surface disruption (level II in b).

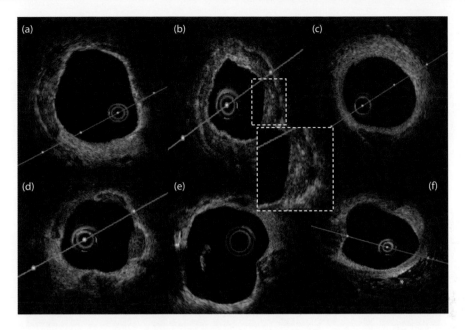

Figure 2.12 Morphological patterns of coronary calcified plaques. These plaques can be readily identified by OCT as signal-poor regions with sharp borders. (a) Eccentric and superficial plaque almost exclusively located in the northwest quadrant. (b) Concentric and superficial plaque surrounding the entire lumen circumference. Note that in the two to four o'clock segment the intimal layer is so thin that it cannot be identified by OCT (below the axial resolution [dashed inbox]. (c) Focal, eccentric, and nonsuperficial calcification at six to nine o'clock. A thick intimal layer lining the calcium plaque is seen. Note that only the southwest quadrant is involved. (d) Focal, concentric, and superficial calcium plaques. Even though the calcium plaques involve all quadrants, distinct nodes of calcium separated by fatty or fibrotic tissue are easily identified. (e) Focal and superficial calcium plaque protruding in the luminal area. It has been suggested that these calcium spikes may be responsible for difficult device navigation or balloon rupture, even in the absence of any perceived significant stenosis. (f) Eccentric and deep calcium plaque (*). Nonsuperficial calcium plaque may be more difficult to identify by OCT due to the limited tissue penetration. The impact of these morphological patterns on the response to plaque-modifying techniques is currently uncertain.

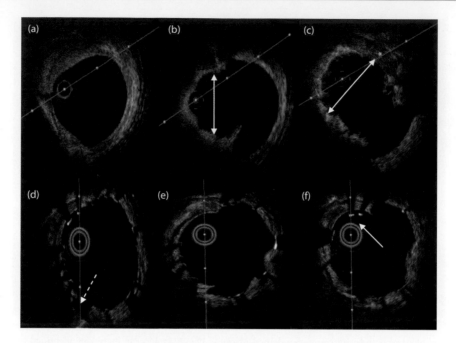

Figure 2.13 Plaque modification by RA with major debulking and channel formation. (a) Eccentric fibrocalcified plaque (nine to twelve o'clock). Note the wire bias (wire in close contact with the vessel wall). (b) After RA with a 1.5 mm burr, major plaque debulking has occurred with a channel formation. The diameter of the channel (solid white double arrow in B) is exactly the same diameter of the burr (1.5 mm). (c) A second passage with a 2 mm burr has resulted in further plaque debulking, superficial calcium plaque denudation (*), and extension of the channel with the same diameter of the second burr (solid white double arrow in c). (d) After stent placement, some segments still showed the presence of the channel behind the struts (white dashed arrow). (e and f) Note also the asymmetric stent expansion and some malapposed struts in the channel site (solid arrow).

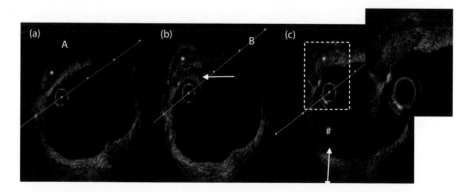

Figure 2.14 Intimal calcium plaque denudation induced by RA. (a) OCT images pre-RA show an eccentric calcium plaque lined by a thick intimal cap. Note the location close to a side branch (one o'clock). (b) Same calcium plaque partially stripped from the intimal cap (arrow) after the first RA 1.25 mm burr passage. (c) Calcium plaque completely denudated after a second and larger 1.5 mm burr passage. Note that the superficial calcium plaque has lost its intimal cap.

2.2.3 Plaque modification after stenting

Currently used techniques of medium- to high-pressure coronary stent implantation frequently create injury on the vessel wall.[9] OCT as a high-resolution imaging technology is very sensitive to luminal abnormalities, and various morphologies of vessel injury after stent implantation have been described, some of which may be underrecognized by angiography or IVUS.[10] Stent edge dissection can be found in up to one-third of cases if OCT is performed routinely. However, only significant tearing at stent edges (Figure 2.15), particularly if angiographically evident, has been associated with adverse events on follow-up.[11] Although readily detected by OCT, the clinical implications and management of other patterns of stent-induced vessel injury (Figures 2.16 through 2.19) are uncertain.[12]

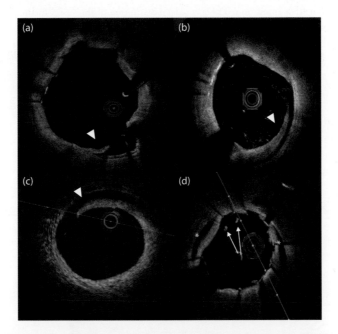

Figure 2.15 (a–c) Flap-type dissection (arrowheads) located at the stent edge (last visible struts). (d) Flap-type dissection sealed by a subexpanded stent. Note the residual wall cavities (*) and intraluminal thrombi (arrows).

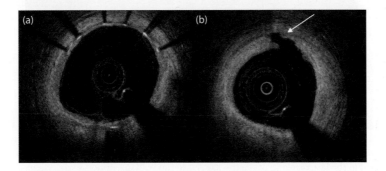

Figure 2.16 Cavity-type stent edge dissection. (a) Distal stent edge positioned over a fibrotic vessel segment. No dissection was apparent from the control angiogram (not shown). (b) OCT shows a cavity-type dissection (arrow) that was left untreated.

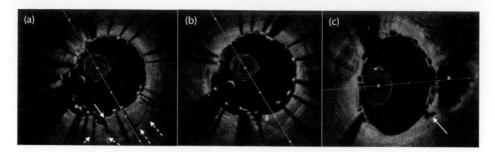

Figure 2.17 (a) Cavity-type intrastent dissection (arrow). Overlapping stents submitted to vigorous high-pressure postdilatation in order to achieve optimal strut apposition. There is a deep disruption of the vessel intima (solid arrow) with associated subintimal hematoma (dashed arrows). Note that a significant malapposition area next to the intrastent dissection persisted despite the postdilatation maneuver. (b) Cross section 0.5 mm proximal to (a) showing the intramural hematoma associated with the dissection (#). (c) Cavity-type dissection associated with a bioabsorbable vascular scaffold at the origin of a collateral branch (*).

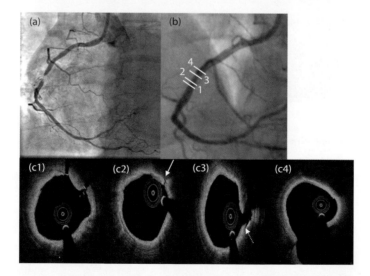

Figure 2.18 Stent edge dissection. (a) Patient with severe stenoses of mid–right coronary artery (RCA) presenting with unstable angina. (b) Good angiographic result after implantation of a 3 × 13 mm stent. Proximal stent edge dissection was not evident. (c1) OCT revealed soft plaque protrusion at the stent border (one o'clock). (c2) Dissection entry point—minimal intimal tear just proximal to the last visible struts (arrow). (c3) Arterial wall disruption with a cavity-type dissection and small associated flap (dashed arrow). (c4) Acute marginal branch ostium used as an anatomic landmark.

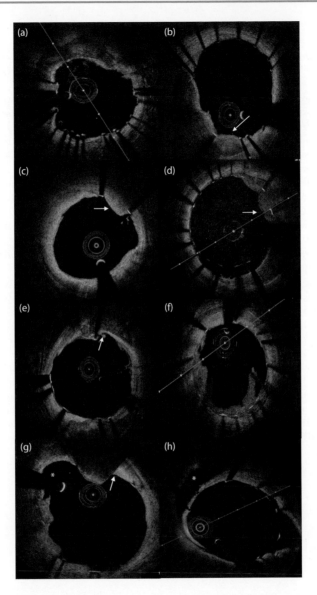

Figure 2.19 Acute effects of stent–tissue interaction. (a) Stent deployed over a superficial eccentric calcified plaque occupying nearly one-third of the vessel circumference (ten to one o'clock), resulting in asymmetric expansion of the stent. (b) Stent implanted over a large eccentric fibrolipidic plaque (six to ten o'clock). There is small localized stent underexpansion with some degree of soft tissue prolapse (arrow). (c) Nonthrombotic tissue prolapse. There is protrusion of tissue between adjacent stent struts without disruption of the continuity of the luminal vessel surface. This has been described to occur in virtually all cases of stent implantation and found to have no immediate clinical implications.[12] (d) Large thrombus lining half of the vessel circumference (twelve to six o'clock) resulting in evident stent undersizing, obvious stent malapposition, and thrombotic tissue prolapse through the struts (arrow). (e) Small intraluminal thrombus (arrow), i.e., luminal mass with dorsal shadowing that is minimally or not connected to the vessel wall. (f) Large luminal thrombus prolapsed through the struts of a stent implanted in a thrombotic saphenous graft. (g) Plaque shifting. Mural thrombus shifted toward the ostium of a collateral branch (*). (h) Stent sealing a vessel rupture induced by an oversized balloon. Note the subintimal cavity (*).

REFERENCES

1. Stone GW et al. Improved procedural results of coronary angioplasty with intravascular ultrasound-guided balloon sizing: The CLOUT Pilot Trial. Clinical Outcomes with Ultrasound Trial (CLOUT) Investigators. *Circulation* 1997;95:2044–52.
2. Tada T et al. Association between tissue characteristics evaluated with optical coherence tomography and mid-term results after paclitaxel-coated balloon dilatation for in-stent restenosis lesions: A comparison with plain old balloon angioplasty. *European Heart Journal* 2014;15:307–15.
3. Costa JR et al. Nonrandomized comparison of coronary stenting under intravascular ultrasound guidance of direct stenting without predilation versus conventional predilation with a semi-compliant balloon versus predilation with a new scoring balloon. *American Journal of Cardiology* 2007;100:812–7.
4. Dahm J et al. Cutting-balloon angioplasty effectively facilitates the interventional procedure and leads to a low rate of recurrent stenosis in ostial bifurcation coronary lesions: A subgroup analysis of the NICECUT multicenter registry. *International Journal of Cardiology* 2008;124:345–50.
5. Kuntz RE et al. The importance of acute luminal diameter in determining restenosis after coronary atherectomy or stenting. *Circulation* 1992;86:1827–35.
6. Colombo A et al. J. Intracoronary stenting without anticoagulation accomplished with intravascular ultrasound guidance. *Circulation* 1995;91:1676–88.
7. Moussa I et al. Subacute stent thrombosis in the era of intravascular ultrasound guided coronary stenting without anticoagulation: Frequency, predictors and clinical outcome. *Journal of the American College of Cardiology* 1997;29:6–12.
8. Henneke KH et al. Impact of target lesion calcification on coronary stent expansion after rotational atherectomy. *American Heart Journal* 1999;137:93–9.
9. Sheris SJ, Canos MR, Weissman NJ. Natural history of intravascular ultrasound-detected edge dissections from coronary stent deployment. *American Heart Journal* 2000;139:59–63.
10. Bouma BE et al. Evaluation of intracoronary stenting by intravascular optical coherence tomography. *Heart* 2003;89:317–20.
11. Chamié D et al. Incidence, predictors, morphological characteristics, and clinical outcomes of stent edge dissections detected by optical coherence tomography. *JACC Cardiovascular Interventions* 2013;6:800–13.
12. Gonzalo N et al. Optical coherence tomography assessment of the acute effects of stent implantation on the vessel wall: A systematic quantitative approach. *Heart* 2009;95:1913–9.

Chapter 3

OCT for plaque modification

Andrejs Erglis

3.1 PLAQUE MODIFICATION BEFORE CORONARY ARTERY STENTING USING CUTTING/SCORING BALLOON

In this chapter, we analyze appropriate atherosclerotic plaque modification before coronary stent implantation using cutting and scoring balloons. Plaque modification prior to stent implantation using cutting and scoring balloons is an essential tool to achieve the best possible result and ensure the long-term safety and efficacy of percutaneous coronary intervention (PCI). Stent expansion remains an important predictor of restenosis and subacute thrombosis, even in the drug-eluting stent (DES) era. Plaque modification with rotational atherectomy or predilatation with a cutting balloon (CB) has been demonstrated to improve stent expansion.[1,2] The risk of suboptimal stent deployment—stent underexpansion, incomplete stent apposition, and incomplete lesion coverage—increases stent restenosis and stent thrombosis.[3,4] Significantly calcified lesions pose a particular challenge to the interventional cardiologist. Calcified coronary lesions are not a homogenous entity, and their response to PCI varies according to the severity of calcification. Severely calcified lesions respond poorly to balloon angioplasty (BA), and when stents are implanted in such lesions, an incomplete and asymmetrical stent expansion occurs in the majority of cases.[5,6] Therefore, adequate plaque modification prior to DES implantation is the key for calcified lesion treatment.[7] The present material was designed to provide data for optical coherence tomography (OCT) imaging in plaque pretreatment and for the assessment of human coronary artery disease and PCI results.

3.2 CUTTING AND SCORING BALLOONS

With regular balloon inflation, the entire balloon surface contacts the vessel wall, disrupting endothelium, nonuniformly compressing plaque, and causing arterial wall damage. An injury produced by a scoring balloon (Figure 3.1) is strictly localized to the scoring sites, sparing most of the endothelium, compressing the plaque, and reducing trauma to the media layer.[8]

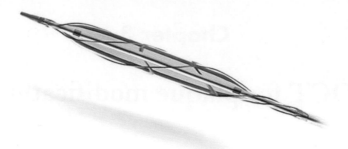

Figure 3.1 AngioSculpt scoring balloon catheter.

CB (Figure 3.2) atherotomes (microsurgical blades) are mounted longitudinally on the outer surface of a balloon and, during expansion, deliver longitudinal incisions in the plaque. The atherotomes deliver a controlled fault line during dilatation to ensure that the crack propagation ensues in an orderly fashion.[9] CB increases vessel lumen diameter in a more controlled fashion, and lower balloon inflation pressure is needed, thus decreasing the risk of a neoproliferative response and restenosis (Figure 3.3). Artery scoring before stent implantation gives almost perfect stent apposition with reduced inflation pressure, even if very long stents are deployed. In bifurcation treatment, it minimizes plaque shifting between the main branch and side branch, thus helping to avoid side branch stenting. Complex coronary lesion interventions in the case of aorto-ostial, small-vessel, and calcified lesions can benefit from pretreatment with scoring devices to minimize balloon slippage, alter calcification, increase artery compliance, and enhance stent deliverability. In our opinion, plaque debulking with directional coronary atherectomy or modification with a scoring device before stent deployment could minimize arterial injury and subsequent neointimal proliferation, and could prevent restenosis formation. We believe that plaque modification with a scoring device or directional coronary atherectomy before stenting minimizes plaque shifting between the main branch and side branch, and thus could help to avoid side branch stenting, as well as give better stent apposition with reduced inflation pressure, even if very long stents are deployed.[10]

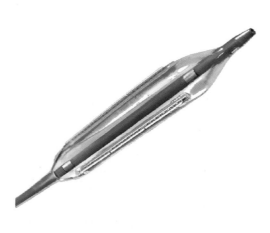

Figure 3.2 CB dilatation device.

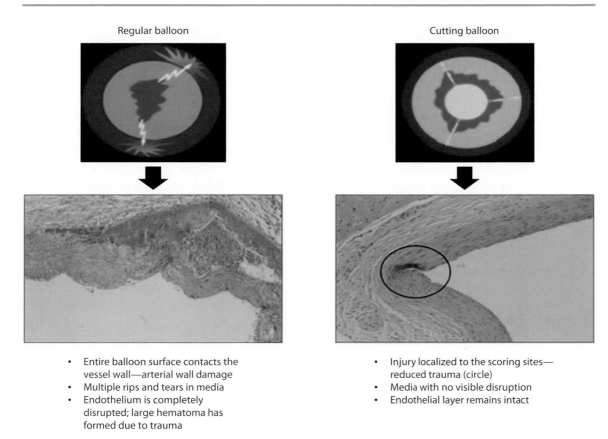

Figure 3.3 Regular balloon and CB: mechanisms of action.

3.3   TRIAL RESULTS WITH CUTTING OR SCORING BALLOON PLAQUE PRETREATMENT

A single-center substudy of Nordic I and Nordic II trials and the Riga bifurcation registry included 556 patients who had undergone PCI of bifurcation lesions. We compared the safety and efficacy of plaque modification with a scoring device prior to main vessel stenting and/or side branch treatment in bifurcation lesions in 209 patients versus 347 patients without plaque modification prior to stenting. Target lesion revascularization (TLR) was lower in the CB group than in the non-CB group 5.3% (n = 11) vs. 11.0% (n = 38), p = 0.021. Target vessel revascularization (TVR) was 8.1% (n = 17) in the CB group vs. 13.8% (n = 48) in the non-CB group (p = 0.056). These outcomes showed that plaque modification using a cutting device before stenting might help to avoid the need for complex stenting and provide a good long-term outcome in patients within the first year postprocedure.[11,12]

The Cutting Balloon Global Randomized Trial was a multicenter, randomized trial on 1238 patients; it tested the hypothesis that "surgical" dilatation using the CB (n = 617) could result in less arterial trauma, fewer dissections, and less frequent restenosis than conventional percutaneous balloon angioplasty (PTCA) (n = 621). The CB group showed no reduction of the binary angiographic restenosis rate at 6 months (31.4% for CB and 30.4% for PTCA, p = 0.75). The secondary endpoints of TLR and major adverse cardiac events (MACEs) after 9 months were also not statistically significant, although freedom from TVR was slightly higher in the CB arm (88.5% vs. 84.6%, log-rank p = 0.04). Five coronary perforations occurred only in the CB arm (0.8% vs. 0%, p = 0.03). The trial showed that CB angioplasty alone was equivalent in safety and efficacy endpoints to PTCA, but did not prove superior.[13]

Iijima et al.[14] conducted a retrospective two-center study that included 327 lesions of small coronaries (less than 2.5 mm in diameter) that were treated by either CB (n = 87), plain old balloon angioplasty (POBA) (n = 130), or bare-metal stent (BMS) implantation (n = 110). At angiographic follow-up, CB angioplasty resulted in less restenosis than the plain balloon or stenting subgroups (31%, 46.5%, and 43.9%, respectively, p = 0.048). MACE (death, myocardial infarction, and TLR) rates at follow-up were significantly lower in the CB angioplasty than the other groups (CB 20.3%, POBA 37.3%, stent 33.3%, p = 0.036).

The Restenosis Reduction by Cutting Balloon Evaluation III (REDUCE III) Japanese prospective randomized multicenter trial enrolled 521 patients who were randomized to CB angioplasty before BMS (CBA-BMS) (n = 260) and to BA before BMS (BA-BMS) (n = 261). The primary endpoint was angiographic restenosis (≥50% diameter stenosis at follow-up by quantitative coronary angiography [QCA]) and subsequent TLR at the 7-month follow-up. Intravascular ultrasound (IVUS)-guided procedures were performed in 279 (54%) patients. Although balloon size prior to stenting was similar between the two groups, the inflated pressure was significantly lower with the CBA group than the BA group. Postprocedural percentage diameter stenosis (%DS) was less in CBA-BMS than in BA-BMS (14.0 ± 5.9% vs. 16.3 ± 6.8%, p < 0.01). %DS at follow-up was subsequently less in CBA-BMS than BA-BMS (32.4 ± 15.1% vs. 35.4 ± 15.3%, p < 0.05), associated with lower rates of restenosis in CBA-BMS than in BA-BMS (11.8% vs. 19.6%, p < 0.05), and associated with less TLR in CBA-BMS than in BA-BMS (9.6% vs. 15.3%, p < 0.05). Patients were also divided into four groups based on the device used before stenting and IVUS use. At follow-up, IVUS-CBA-BMS had a significantly lower restenosis rate (6.6%) than angio-CBA-BMS (17.9%), IVUS-BA-BMS (19.8%), and angio-BA-BMS (18.2%, p < 0.05). In addition, multivariate analyses indicated that the use of BA was an independent predictor for stent restenosis at follow-up. The results of this study strongly suggested that use of appropriate plaque modification and IVUS guidance during intervention significantly increases the acute and postprocedural results of angioplasty.[15]

Nonrandomized comparison by De Ribamar Costa et al. includes 224 consecutive patients with 299 *de novo* lesions treated with one DES in a nonrandomized fashion. Patients were assigned to direct stenting without predilatation (n = 145), a conventional semicompliant balloon (n = 117), or predilatation with the AngioSculpt® scoring balloon (n = 37). The primary goal was to assess stent expansion, defined as the ratio of IVUS-measured minimum stent diameter (MSD) and area (MSA) to the predicted stent diameter (PSD) and area (PSA). Patients pretreated with AngioSculpt had significantly better stent expansion, reaching 88% ± 18% of the predicted final stent area (p < 0.001). No significant difference was found between patients pretreated with the conventional semicompliant balloon and those with direct stent deployment (76% ± 13% vs. 76% ± 10%, p = 0.8). Only 0.6% of direct stent patients and 5% of stents placed after conventional predilatation achieved PSD, as opposed to 18.9% of stents pretreated with AngioSculpt (p < 0.001). The MSA/PSA and MSD/PSD ratios were larger with AngioSculpt predilatation, and a greater percentage of stents had a final MSA of >5.0 mm^2. The main conclusion of this study is that DESs are commonly underexpanded and fail to achieve even minimum standards of stent expansion that may lead to DES-related adverse events. Notably, conventional balloon predilatation does not improve the final stent expansion compared with direct stenting.[16]

3.4 PATIENT'S CLINICAL CASES USING CUTTING AND SCORING PLAQUE PRETREATMENT

We analyze three clinical cases using cutting and scoring balloons in plaque pretreatment and OCT guidance for optimal stent deployment. OCT imaging was performed after intracoronary injection of nitroglycerin

(100–200 μg) before and after CB pretreatment, and after stent implantation. Frequency-domain OCT (FD-OCT) was performed with a 2.7 F OCT catheter (Dragonfly imaging catheter, LightLab Imaging, Westford, Massachusetts), and blood clearance was achieved by nondiluted iodine contrast injection at rates of 3–5 mL/s for a total volume of 10–20 mL/pullback. Images were acquired with an automated pullback at a rate of 1 mm/s for time-domain OCT (TD-OCT) and 20 mm/s for FD-OCT.

3.4.1 First clinical case

An 80-year-old woman was admitted with severe angina during physical activity. She had a history of previous PCI of the left main (LM). From cardiovascular risk factors, she had well-controlled arterial hypertension, dyslipidemia, non-insulin-dependent diabetes mellitus, and a positive family history. An exercise stress test showed ischemic changes in the left ventricle anterior wall. The patient was chronically treated with aspirin (ASA), beta-blockers, calcium channel blockers, angiotensin-converting-enzyme (ACE) inhibitors, nitrates, and statins. Angiography showed a tight bifurcation lesion of >75% in the left anterior descending artery/diagonal (LAD/D) (Medina classification 1,1,1) (Figure 3.4). Preintervention OCT showed heavily calcified eccentric stenosis in the LAD (Figure 3.5) and fibrotic tissue with lipid pools in the diagonal branch (Figure 3.6). Plaque modification was performed with a 2.5 × 10 mm AngioSculpt balloon in the main branch (Figure 3.7) and side branch (Figure 3.8). DES implantation in the LAD across the diagonal branch was followed by postdilatation with an noncompliant (NC) balloon. Postintervention OCT showed the optimal final result (Figure 3.9). The diagonal branch was left with thrombolysis in myocardial infarction (TIMI) 3 flow. The patient was symptom-free on optimal medicament treatment at the 1-year follow-up (Figure 3.10).

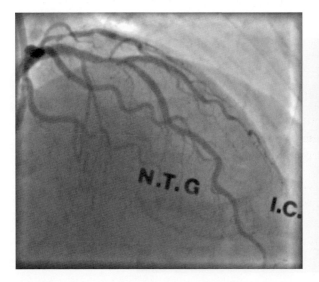
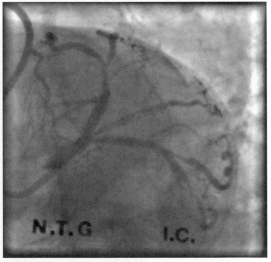

Figure 3.4 Angiography of the LAD/Diagonal bifurcation stenosis. Angiography demonstrates 75% stenosis in the LAD and the diagonal branch at the bifurcation. (Medina classification 1,1,1). NTG, nitroglycerine; IC, intracoronary.

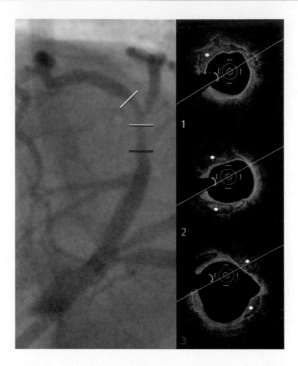

Figure 3.5 OCT imaging before intervention in the LAD lesion. Three OCT cross section images of an eccentric calcified plaque (white asterisks, calcium) on the right, with corresponding angiography image on the left.

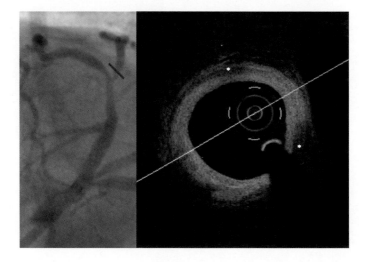

Figure 3.6 OCT imaging before intervention in the diagonal branch. OCT of the diagonal branch shows fibrotic tissue with lipid pools (white asterisks) on the right. Angiography image on the left shows the OCT cross-sectional image acquisition place, marked in red.

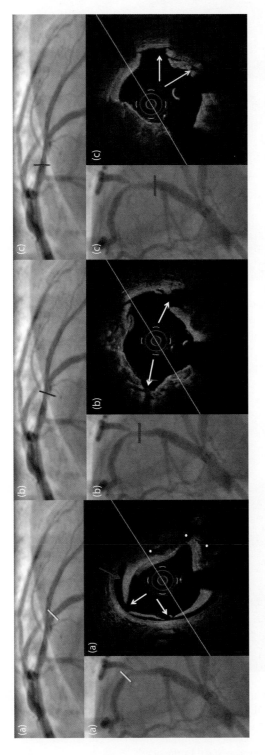

Figure 3.7 (a–c). **OCT imaging after plaque pretreatment in the LAD with AngioSculpt scoring balloon.** (a) OCT cross-sectional segment view (angiography images, yellow lines) after the AngioSculpt balloon in the distal part of the LAD lesion. OCT image shows atheromatous plaque disruption in the vessel wall after the scoring balloon (white arrows) with lumen dissection (red arrow). There are calcium cracks with intraluminal hematomas (white asterisks). (b) OCT cross-sectional segment view (angiography images, red lines) after the AngioSculpt balloon in the middle part of the LAD lesion. OCT image shows the same atheromatous plaque disruption in the vessel wall (white arrows) with lumen dissections. There is some calcium part that is not pretreated well—calcium is not ruptured. In the longitudinal angiographic image, there are dissections after the scoring balloon in this particular segment. (c) OCT cross-sectional segment view (angiography images, red lines) after the AngioSculpt balloon in the proximal part of the LAD lesion. In the OCT image, the white arrow shows the complete plaque cut, but the yellow arrow shows only a partial one.

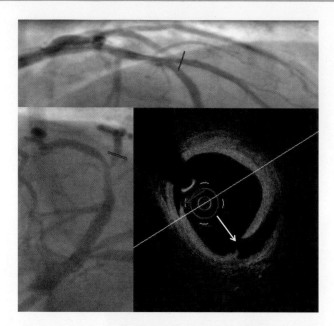

Figure 3.8 OCT imaging after plaque pretreatment in the diagonal branch with AngioSculpt scoring balloon. OCT cross-sectional segment view (angiography images, red lines) after the AngioSculpt balloon in the proximal part of the diagonal branch. In the OCT image, the white arrow shows a complete plaque cut and the red arrow a partial one.

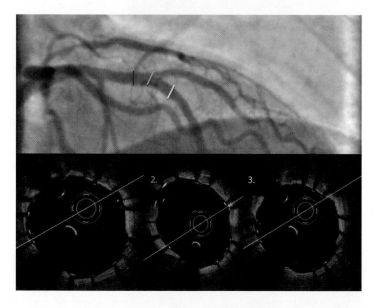

Figure 3.9 OCT imaging after stent implantation in the LAD and postdilatation with NC balloon. OCT cross-sectional views of the LAD poststenting (3.0 × 15 mm DES at 11 bar). Left to right: Proximal to distal, every cross-sectional segment is marked in a different color. OCT images show complete lesion coverage with good strut apposition to the vessel wall. There are no signs of malapposition or plaque protrusion after postdilatation with the NC balloon, 3.0 × 12 mm at 18 bar. All dissections that were made by the scoring balloon were covered by the stent.

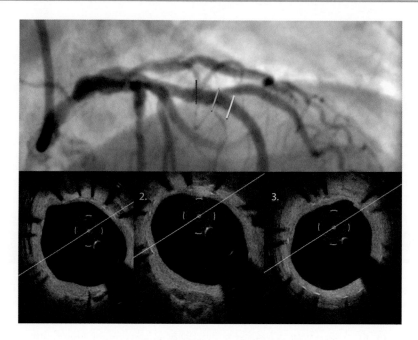

Figure 3.10 OCT imaging of the LAD at 12-month follow-up. OCT cross-sectional views of the LAD at the 12-month follow-up. Left to right: Proximal to distal, every cross-sectional segment is marked in a different color. OCT images show complete strut covering with neointima.

3.4.2 Second clinical case

A 70-year-old woman with stable angina grade 2 was planned for elective PCI. From cardiovascular risk factors, she had well-controlled arterial hypertension and dyslipidemia. She was chronically treated with ASA, calcium channel blockers, an ACE inhibitor, and statins.

Angiography showed a bifurcation lesion of >75% in the LAD/D (Medina classification 1,1,0) (Figure 3.11). Preintervention OCT for the LAD lesion preprocedure was done (Figure 3.12). We performed scoring balloon pretreatment in the LAD lesion (2.5 × 15 mm at 8 bar) following OCT (Figure 3.13a–c). After scoring balloon pretreatment, a DES was implanted (3.0 × 23 mm at 11 bar), and postdilatation with an NC balloon was done (3.5 × 15 mm at 13 bar), as well as OCT final control (Figure 3.14). The diagonal branch was not treated, but strut opening was performed with a 2.0 × 8 mm balloon. At the 12-month follow-up, the patient was asymptomatic without angina complaints (Figure 3.15).

3.4.3 Third clinical case

A 61-year-old woman with stable angina grade 3 was planned for elective PCI for a LAD/D bifurcation lesion. From cardiovascular risk factors, she had arterial hypertension, dyslipidemia, and previous myocardial infarction with urgent PCI for right coronary artery (RCA). She was a smoker for more than 20 years. Angiography showed a bifurcation lesion of >75% in the LAD/D with severe stenosis in the diagonal branch ostium (Medina classification 1,0,1) (Figure 3.16). Preintervention OCT was done for the LAD lesion preprocedure (Figure 3.17) and for the diagonal branch ostium (Figure 3.18). The CB pretreatment done in the LAD and diagonal branch (3.25 × 10 mm at 6 bar and 2.5 × 6 mm at 6 bar) and after OCT controls for both branches (Figure 3.19) for the LAD and (Figure 3.20) for the diagonal branch. After plaque pretreatment,

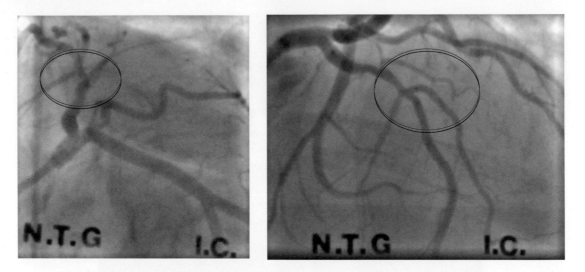

Figure 3.11 Angiography of the LAD/Diagonal bifurcation stenosis. Angiography view of the LAD/D bifurcation lesion with more than 75% stenosis (red marked). Medina classification 1,1,0. NTG, nitroglycerine; IC, intracoronary.

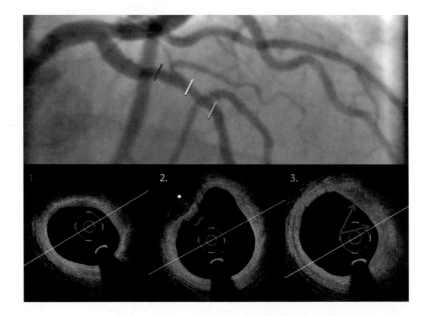

Figure 3.12 Pre-procedure OCT of the LAD bifurcation lesion. Angiography view and OCT cross-sectional views of the LAD lesion preprocedure. White asterisk, calcium plaque. The distal cross-sectional image (red arrows) shows fibrotic and lipid pool plaque.

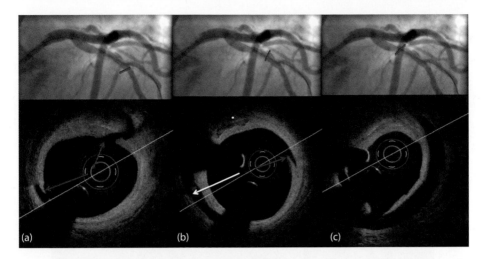

Figure 3.13 (a–c) OCT of the LAD bifurcation lesion after scoring balloon pretreatment. (a) Angiography and OCT view after scoring balloon pretreatment at the distal part of the LAD lesion (red mark on angiographic image shows OCT cross-sectional position). OCT image shows complete plaque cut (red arrows). (b) Angiography and OCT view after scoring balloon pretreatment at the middle part of the LAD lesion (red mark on angiographic image shows OCT cross-sectional position). OCT shows incomplete plaque cut (red arrow)—calcium part is still not cut (white asterisk)—and intramural hematoma (white arrow and red mark on angiographic view). (c) Angiography and OCT view after scoring balloon pretreatment at the proximal part of the LAD lesion (red mark on angiographic image shows OCT cross-sectional position). OCT shows a good plaque pretreatment result with complete plaque disruption.

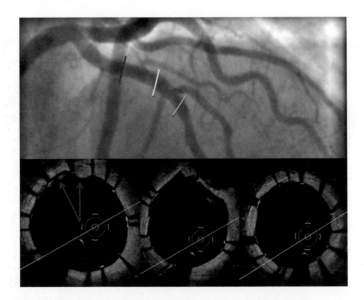

Figure 3.14 Angiography and OCT after stent implantation in the LAD lesion. OCT cross-sectional views of the LAD lesion poststenting. Left to right: Proximal to distal, every cross-sectional segment is marked in a different color. OCT images show complete lesion coverage with good strut apposition to the vessel wall. At the proximal cross section view, OCT reveals small intraluminal plaque protrusion through the stent struts (red arrows).

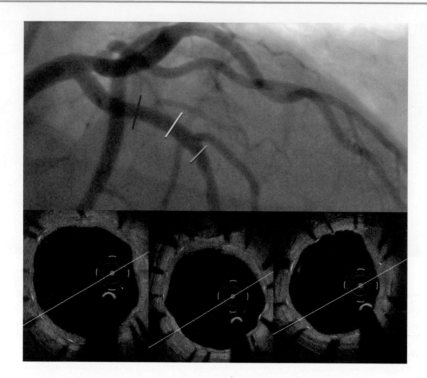

Figure 3.15 Angiography and OCT 12-months after stent implantation in the LAD lesion. Angiography and OCT views at the 12-month poststenting of the LAD lesion. Left to right: Proximal to distal, every cross-sectional segment is marked in a different color. OCT images show complete stent strut coverage.

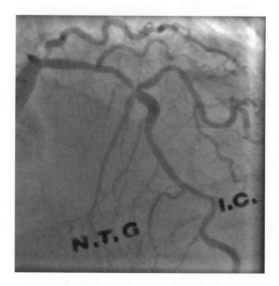

Figure 3.16 Angiography of the LAD/Diagonal bifurcation. Angiography view of the LAD bifurcation with a large diagonal branch. Medina classification 1,0,1. NTG, nitroglycerine; IC, intracoronary.

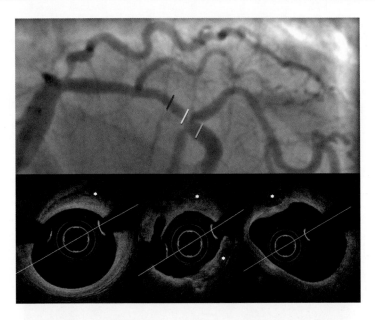

Figure 3.17 Angiography and OCT before intervention in the LAD/Diagonal bifurcation. Angiography and OCT views of the LAD lesion preprocedure. Left to right: Proximal to distal, every cross-sectional segment is marked in a different color. OCT images show mixed lipid pull plaque with calcification (white asterisks).

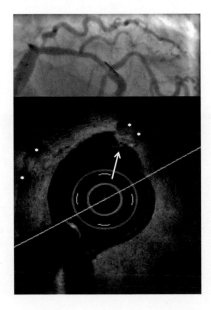

Figure 3.18 Angiography and OCT views pre-procedure of the diagonal branch ostium. Angiography and OCT views of the diagonal branch ostium preprocedure. OCT image shows very tight lesion with rich lipid pool plaque, some calcification (white asterisks), and signs of plaque rupturing or ulceration (white arrow).

it was decided to treat bifurcation with two stents using a crush technique (3.0 × 23 mm at 15 bar in the LAD and 2.8 × 8 mm at 15 bar in the diagonal branch). Postdilatation with an NC balloon was done in the main branch (3.5 × 15 mm at 15 bar), and OCT final control was done at the LAD (Figure 3.21). The diagonal branch was dissected after stent implantation with TIMI 1 flow. At the 10-month follow-up, the patient was asymptomatic without angina complaints with a good result by OCT (Figure 3.22). The diagonal branch was fully opened with TIMI 3.

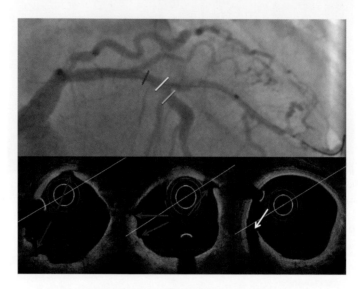

Figure 3.19 Angiography and OCT views of the LAD lesion post cutting balloon pretreatment. Angiography and OCT views of the LAD lesion post-CB plaque pretreatment. Left to right: Proximal to distal, every cross-sectional segment is marked in a different color. OCT images show complete plaque cut (white arrow) and incomplete cuts (red arrows).

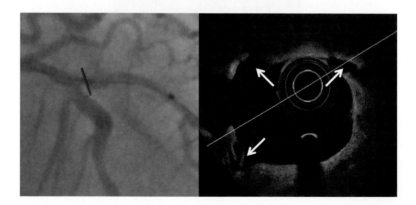

Figure 3.20 Angiography and OCT view of the diagonal branch ostial lesion post cutting balloon pretreatment. Angiography and OCT views of the diagonal branch lesion post-CB plaque pretreatment. OCT image shows completely cut plaque (white arrows).

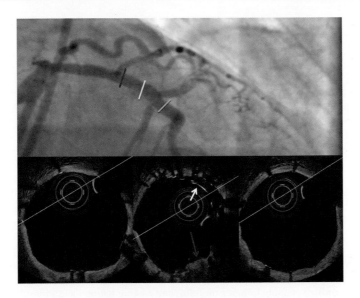

Figure 3.21 Angiography and OCT views of the LAD lesion poststenting. Angiography and OCT views of the LAD lesion poststenting. Left to right: Proximal to distal, every cross-sectional segment is marked in a different color. OCT images show complete stent strut coverage and double stent strut layer (white arrow), with intraluminal plaque protrusion through the stent struts (red arrow).

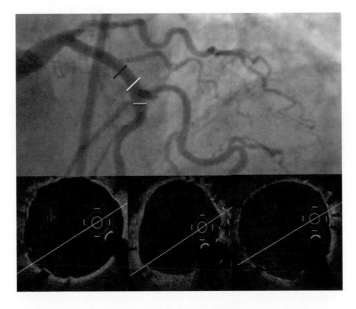

Figure 3.22 Angiography and OCT views of LAD lesion at 10-month follow up. Angiography and OCT views of the LAD lesion poststenting at the 10-month follow-up. Left to right: Proximal to distal, every cross-sectional segment is marked in a different color. OCT images show complete stent strut coverage.

REFERENCES

1. Serruys PW et al. A comparison of balloon-expandable-stent implantation with balloon angioplasty in patients with coronary artery disease. *New England Journal of Medicine* 1994;331(8):489–95.
2. Stone GW et al. A polymer-based, paclitaxel-eluting stent in patients with coronary artery disease. *New England Journal of Medicine* 2004;350(3):221–31.
3. Cook S et al. Incomplete stent apposition and very late stent thrombosis after drug-eluting stent implantation. *Circulation* 2007;115(18):2426–34.
4. Fujii K et al. Stent underexpansion and residual reference segment stenosis are related to stent thrombosis after sirolimus-eluting stent implantation: An intravascular ultrasound study. *Journal of the American College of Cardiology* 2005;45(7):995–8.
5. Ellis SG et al. Coronary morphologic and clinical determinants of procedural outcome with angioplasty for multivessel coronary disease. Implications for patient selection. Multivessel Angioplasty Prognosis Study Group. *Circulation* 1990;82:1193–202.
6. Tanigawa J, Barlis P, Di Mario C. Heavily calcified coronary lesions preclude strut apposition despite high pressure balloon dilatation and rotational atherectomy: In-vivo demonstration with optical coherence tomography. *Circulation Journal* 2008;72:157–60.
7. Zhe Tang et al. Cutting-balloon angioplasty before drug-eluting stent implantation for the treatment of severely calcified coronary lesions. *Journal of Geriatric Cardiology* 2014;11:44–9.
8. Okura H et al. Mechanisms of acute lumen gain following cutting balloon angioplasty in calcified and noncalcified lesions: An intravascular ultrasound study. *Catheterization and Cardiovascular Interventions* 2002;57(4):429–36.
9. Ajani AE et al. Clinical utility of the cutting balloon. *Journal of Invasive Cardiology* 2001;13(7):554–7.
10. Andrejs Erglis et al. Importance of plaque modification before coronary artery stenting. *EMJ Interventional Cardiology* 2013;1:64–9.
11. Tsuchikane E et al. Pre-drug-eluting stent debulking of bifurcated coronary lesions. *Journal of the American College of Cardiology* 2007;50:1941–45.
12. Erglis A. Arterial scoring: Cosmetic or curative. Presented at the Transcatheter Cardiovascular Therapeutics Meeting, San Francisco, September 21–25, 2009.
13. Mauri L et al. Cutting balloon angioplasty for the prevention of restenosis: Results of the Cutting Balloon Global Randomized Trial. *American Journal of Cardiology* 2002;90(10):1079–83.
14. Iijima R et al. Cutting balloon angioplasty is superior to balloon angioplasty or stent implantation for small coronary artery disease. *Coronary Artery Disease* 2004;15(7):435–40.
15. Ozaki Y et al. Impact of cutting balloon angioplasty (CBA) prior to bare metal stenting on restenosis. *Circulation* 2007;71(1):1–8.
16. De Ribamar Costa J et al. Nonrandomized comparison of coronary stenting under intravascular ultrasound guidance of direct stenting without predilation versus conventional predilation with a semi-compliant balloon versus predilation with a new scoring balloon. *American Journal of Cardiology* 2007;100(5):812–7.

Chapter 4

OCT for stent optimization

Satoko Tahara, Yusuke Fujino, and Sunao Nakamura

4.1 INTRODUCTION

Intravascular optical coherence tomography (OCT) is a modality for visualizing the vessel lumen during contrast injection, while angiography shows the vessel lumen as an x-ray shadow image created by contrast. Luminal information provided by OCT is not affected by projection angle or vessel morphology, such as angulations, calcification, and diffuse plaque distribution, and lesion severity can thus be accurately assessed with OCT. Furthermore, OCT is superior to angiography in evaluating calcium distribution and plaque tissue characteristics. Previous intravascular ultrasound (IVUS) studies[1–4] indicate that angiographic success cannot always be linked with optimal stent expansion, so complementary intravascular imaging information provided by OCT (in place of IVUS) is also useful to determine stent size, accomplish optimal stent deployment, and confirm stent apposition without edge dissection and large residual plaque at the stent edges. In this chapter, we discuss how to use OCT during PCI to accomplish optimal stenting.

4.2 UTILIZATION OF OCT FOR VESSEL PREPARATION

4.2.1 Thrombectomy

Aspiration thrombectomy during acute myocardial infarction is considered to be beneficial in reducing major adverse cardiac events (MACEs), including mortality, at 6–12 months compared with conventional primary PCI alone.[5] Residual thrombus burden in acute coronary syndrome may cause acquired stent malapposition at late follow-up.[6] Furthermore, thrombus around a ruptured plaque frequently prevents the acquisition of luminal surface information. OCT can easily evaluate the thrombus occupying the lumen, even that which is not clearly defined on angiography (Figure 4.1). OCT measurement of the thrombus burden at primary PCI is feasible,[7] and thus OCT can also be used to assess whether manual aspiration has been performed successfully. Moreover, following OCT after successful thrombus aspiration, the treatment strategy might be changed if the etiology of the thrombus is found to be plaque erosion instead of plaque rupture.[8]

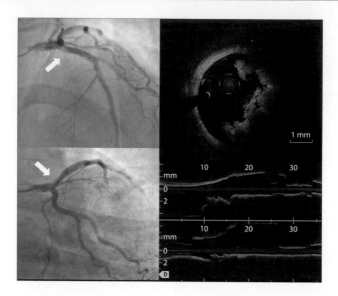

Figure 4.1 An acute coronary syndrome patient presenting with ambiguous angiography (left panels) at assessment of the significantly stenosed target lesion. An OCT pullback image appreciated the large thrombus associated with ruptured plaque in the most proximal left anterior descending artery (right panels).

4.2.2 Calcium modification using rotational atherectomy or cutting balloon

Stent placement in calcified lesions can result in stent underexpansion, malapposition, and procedural complications. High-speed rotational atherectomy is useful for calcium modification that allows a balloon catheter to be fully dilated, making optimal stent expansion possible. OCT can quickly assess both calcium distribution and the achieved modification of ring calcium and/or protruding calcium by rotational atherectomy (Figure 4.2). As an additional tool, the use of cutting balloon inflation within a calcified lesion before stenting is also helpful for overcoming calcific restraint, which can be unresponsive to high-pressure inflation with noncompliant balloons (Figure 4.3).

4.3 OCT FOR DEFINING STENT LENGTH AND DIAMETER

4.3.1 Defining lumen profile

There are few studies investigating the feasibility of OCT guidance for PCI. One multicenter trial, which compared the clinical outcomes of angiography-guided PCI versus an OCT-guided strategy in patients with stable angina, showed that the group treated with OCT had a lower rate of cardiac death and revascularization at 1 year.[9] OCT is adequate for assessing stent deployment based on lumen criteria. Stent sizing should be performed based on reference lumen diameters with minimal plaques. Utilizing the Ilumien™ Optis™ Lumen Profile (St. Jude Medical, St. Paul, Minnesota, a commercially available automatic lumen detection system, the appropriate stent length and diameter can be easily determined (Figure 4.4). In cases with a tight stenosis that inhibits blood clearance, predilation before OCT image acquisition is recommended to acquire images for the lumen profile. Additional manual lumen correction is sometimes required for blurred lumen

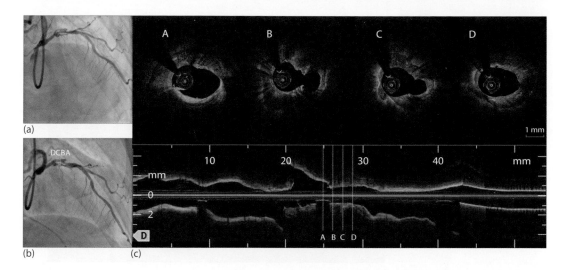

Figure 4.2 Case 1. OCT during rotational atherectomy. A 66-year-old female who had a past history of Kawasaki disease presented with stable angina and underwent coronary angiography, which showed the aneurysm and the proximal adjacent stenosis in the proximal left anterior descending artery. An OCT catheter was unable to cross the tightest lesion at preprocedure (a). The ring calcium was successfully ablated with a 1.75 mm burr after a 1.5 mm burr (b), so that the OCT catheter could easily proceed into the vessel to evaluate the ablated proximal calcified lesion (c).

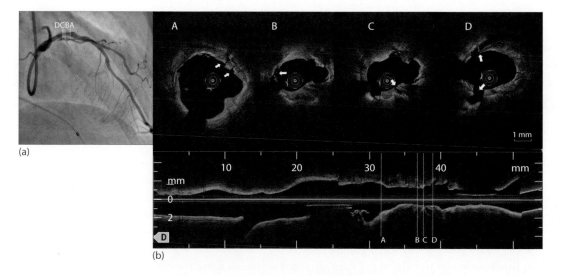

Figure 4.3 Case 1. OCT evaluation after cutting balloon. Angiogram (a) and OCT pullback (b) images after cutting balloon inflation from Case 1. The use of 3.0 × 10 mm cutting balloon inflation within a calcified lesion after rotational atherectomy was also helpful to overcome calcific restraint. White arrows indicate dissections created by cutting balloon inflation.

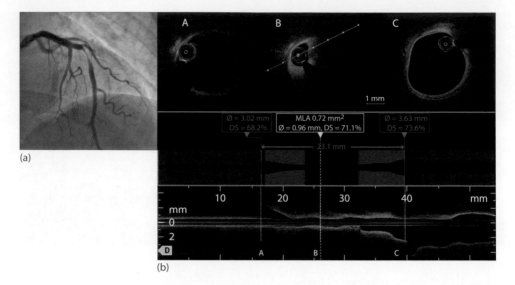

Figure 4.4 Ilumien Optis Lumen Profile. (a) Angiogram before the procedure. (b) OCT lumen profile image: (A) distal reference, (B) minimal lumen area, and (C) proximal reference.

contours, i.e., lumens with residual blood, large side branches, and noncircular geometry when operating the automatic detection algorithm.

4.3.2   Screening for unstable plaques

OCT is useful to screen for unstable plaques that exist in the target vessel when deciding the stenting zone. To prevent edge restenosis at late follow-up, locating stent edges on unstable plaques should be avoided. Incomplete stent coverage of unstable plaques appears to be associated with an increased risk for post-procedural myocardial infarction.[10] Unstable plaques with mild stenoses that can be missed with angiographic assessment are easily detected by OCT. Those located close to the culprit lesion are recommended to be sealed together with a longer stent (Figure 4.5).

4.3.3   Defining the best stent landing zone

As described previously, the segment with minimal plaque should be chosen as a reference segment. The lower penetration of OCT frequently precludes the measurement of the vessel diameter (media to media) at segments with a large amount of plaque, which is easily performed at reference segments with a small amount of fibrotic or calcified plaque. In such cases, the determination of the appropriate stent diameter is straightforward. Reference segments with a relatively large amount of plaque may be chosen when diffuse plaque is distributed through the entire vessel in particular patient subsets, such as diabetics. For such cases, the angiogram coregistration function would be helpful to locate reference segments along the coronary angiogram (Figure 4.6). The appropriate stent diameter is usually the same as the reference lumen diameter to avoid plaque injuries at stent edges, but might be larger than the reference lumen diameter in tapered vessels. To minimize plaque injury at stent edges, selection of oversized stents or initial deployment at higher pressures is discouraged.

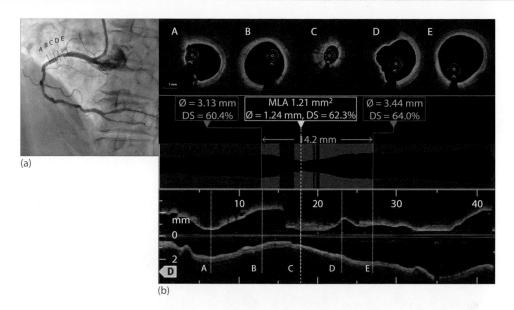

Figure 4.5 Easy detection of unstable plaques, i.e., thin-cap fibroatheromas using OCT. Unstable plaque that exists close to the minimal lumen site of the target lesion could be simultaneously sealed with a longer stent. (a) Angiogram at preprocedure. (b) OCT pullback image. A thin-cap fibroatheroma (A) existed near another thin-cap fibroatheroma (D) associated with the minimal lumen site (C) beyond the originally selected distal reference (B). (E) Proximal reference.

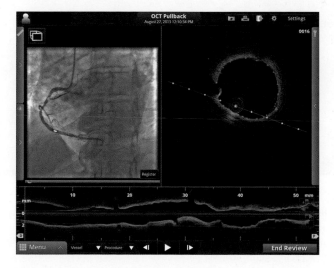

Figure 4.6 Optis integrated system with angio coregistration. A side-by-side view of angiography and OCT with a coregistration function to "map" culprit lesions would make stent selection and deployment much easier.

4.4 OCT FOR SIDE BRANCH PROTECTION

Protection of the side branch for large perfusion territories is mandatory at the time of bifurcation stenting. OCT is useful to predict side branch patency after crossover stenting. The longitudinal OCT pullback image appreciates the location and luminal size of the side branch, as well as the angulation between the main branch and side branch. This information allows us to predict whether the carina shift may compromise side branch patency (Figure 4.7). Plaque distribution at the side branch ostium, side branch size, vessel tortuosity, and calcium distribution along the main branch opposite the side branch[11] may influence side branch patency. Since the imaged vessels always appear straightened on OCT longitudinal images, expectation of side branch

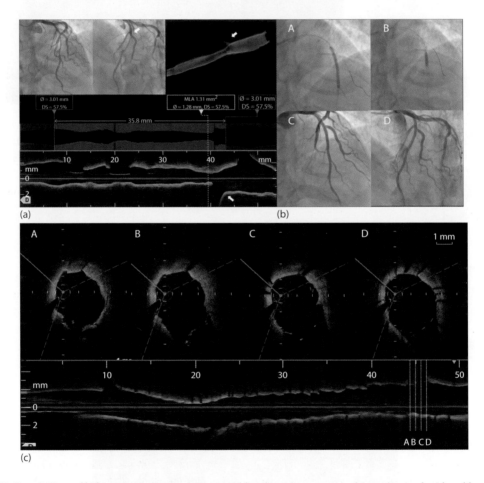

Figure 4.7 Case 2. Case of bifurcation stenting. A 54-year-old male with current smoking presented with stable angina and underwent coronary angiography, which showed a diffuse stenosis in the mid–left anterior descending artery, with the large diagonal branch arising from the white arrow (a, upper left panels). Right upper panel is three-dimensional OCT image. On the OCT longitudinal image, at preprocedure (a, lower panel), although the carina shift was expected to occur after crossover stenting, the large lumen size of the side branch ostium with minimal plaque seemed adequate to keep side branch patency from being compromised. After direct stenting of 3.0 × 38 mm Xience Prime (b, A), followed by postdilation with a 3.5 × 12 mm noncompliant balloon (b, B), the side branch remained angiographically patent (b, C and D). OCT after stenting demonstrated a carina shift that did not compromise diagonal branch patency (c).

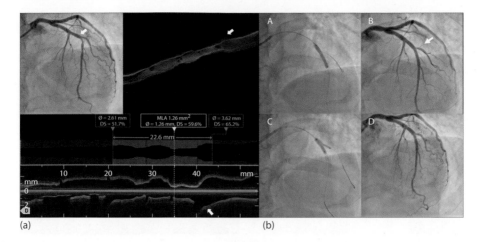

Figure 4.8 Case 3. Another bifurcation stenting case where a carina shift occurred after crossover stenting, which necessitates kissing balloon inflation. A 74-year-old male who presented positive on an exercise test underwent coronary angiography (a, left upper panel). Although a longitudinal OCT image at preprocedure (a, lower panel) showed a similar side branch appearance as Case 2, the carina shift pinched the side branch patency after crossover stenting. (b) A, direct stenting of 3.5 × 23 mm Xience Prime; B, pinched diagonal branch; C, kissing balloon dilation with 3.0 × 15 mm and 2.0 × 15 mm noncompliant balloons; and D, final angiogram.

patency after crossover stenting might be misinformed without consideration of the original angiographic appearance of the target vessel (Figure 4.8).

4.4.1   OCT after stent deployment

Suboptimal stent deployment, including stent underexpansion, incomplete stent apposition, edge dissection, and incomplete lesion coverage, has been reported to be a potent IVUS predictor of stent restenosis and stent thrombosis.[12–14] These unfavorable conditions can be recognized by OCT, allowing for correction by additional procedures.

4.4.2   Stent malapposition

Lumen conditions after stenting can be evaluated using the Ilumien Optis Lumen Profile system that detects the minimal lumen area site after stenting automatically (Figure 4.9). Automatic stent detection is not yet commercially available; therefore, manual measurement is currently necessary to determine malapposition. Struts are defined as malapposed when the distance between the strut and the luminal surface is greater than the sum of the strut and polymer thickness for a drug-eluting stent and the strut alone for a bare-metal stent. While acute incomplete stent apposition after stent deployment correlates with late incomplete neointimal coverage, the malapposition will frequently be resolved at late follow-up when the distance between the strut and lumen surface is less than 380 μm, as demonstrated by a recent OCT study using everolimus-eluting stents (EESs).[15] This finding is longer than the defined malapposition distance of EESs. Malapposition frequently occurs in tapered vessels, overlapped stents, eccentric vessels (noncircular lumen geometry), coronary aneurysms, and the presence of superficial calcium (Figure 4.10). Postdilation with a noncompliant balloon is usually effective for correction of malapposition.

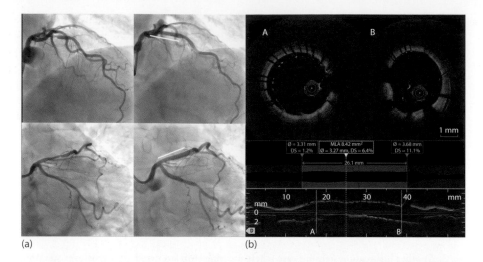

Figure 4.9 Malapposition detected immediately after stenting (3.5 × 23 mm Xience Xpedition) in the proximal left anterior descending artery. (a) Preprocedural (left) and postprocedural (right) angiograms are shown. White lines indicate stented segments. (b) On the OCT image after stenting, malapposed struts were observed in the flared segment (A) and bifurcation (B).

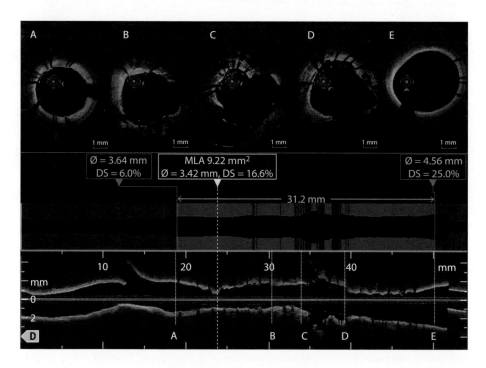

Figure 4.10 Case 1. Acute malappositions associated with several etiologies. OCT images immediately after stenting (3.5 × 28 mm Xience Prime). (A) Satisfactory apposition at the distal edge. (B–D) Malapposition due to noncircular lumen geometry associated with superficial calcium and aneurismal vessel geometry. (E) Malapposition at the most proximal segment of the tapered vessel.

The higher resolution of OCT makes evaluation of stent apposition at side branches much easier. After the kissing balloon technique, OCT for side branch imaging is useful to assess the strut apposition in cases with either single-stent or two-stent implantation (Figure 4.11). A recent study that evaluated the feasibility of OCT for side branch wire recrossing before the kissing balloon technique showed that OCT use was associated with a lower incidence of malapposition around the side branch ostium.[16] The impact of this lower incidence on clinical outcomes has not yet been confirmed.

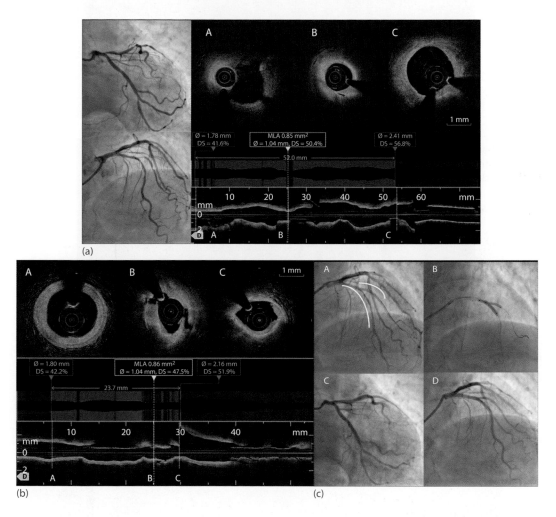

Figure 4.11 Case 4. OCT evaluation during systematic use of two stent mini-crush techniques in the left anterior descending artery (LAD). An 82-year old male who presented with angina pectoris underwent coronary angiography, which showed true bifurcation stenoses (a, left panels). Diffusely distributed plaque along the main LAD (a, right panels) and diagonal branch (b) was observed on preprocedure OCT. Mini-crush stenting was performed according to OCT measurements using 2.75 × 30 mm and 2.75 × 26 mm Endeavor for the main LAD and 2.5 × 26 mm for the diagonal branch (c, A). White lines indicate stented segments. Final kissing balloon inflation was performed with 3.0 × 15 mm and 2.25 × 20 mm noncompliant balloons for the main LAD and diagonal branch, respectively (c, B). Final angiograms are also shown (c, C and D).

(Continued)

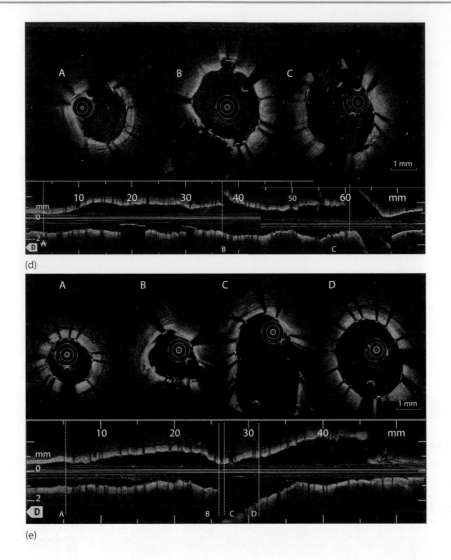

(d)

(e)

Figure 4.11 (Continued) Case 4. OCT evaluation during systematic use of two stent mini-crush techniques in the left anterior descending artery (LAD). Final OCT pullbacks from both the main LAD and side branch showed favorable expansion at the ostiums of both the main LAD (d) and diagonal branch (e).

4.4.3 Stent underexpansion

There is a general agreement that gross stent underexpansion is associated with a higher subsequent risk of in-stent restenosis and/or thrombosis. Calcification is one of the causes of stent underexpansion that significantly increases the subsequent risks of restenosis and/or stent thrombosis. Large plaque burden is another etiology of underexpansion. OCT enables the detection of angiographically unrecognized underexpansion to be corrected by additional postdilation (Figure 4.12). Eccentric calcium distribution at the site of underexpansion should be carefully treated with gradual increases of inflation pressure during postdilation; otherwise, the higher pressures may increase the risk of coronary perforation.

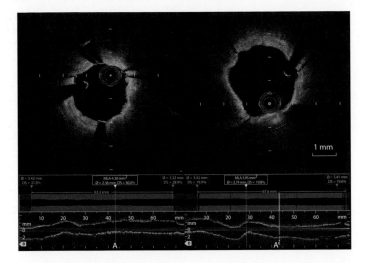

Figure 4.12 Underexpansion after stenting (left) was resolved after postdilation with a 3.5 × 13 mm noncompliant balloon (right).

4.4.4 Edge dissection

OCT can be used to determine stent edge dissections. In a recent study, the overall incidence of OCT-detected edge dissection was 37.8%, of which 84% were not apparent on angiography.[17] In the same study, although additional stenting was performed in 22.6% of all dissections, MACE at 1 year was similar regardless of dissections. Although no numerical index for dissection dimensions that necessitate additional stenting exists, longer dissections with larger dimensions that may cause flow limitation of the target vessel should be shielded (Figure 4.13). Furthermore, large dissections in lipid-rich plaques that may be associated with restenosis should also be corrected. Smaller, thin dissections can be left without additional stenting (Figure 4.14).

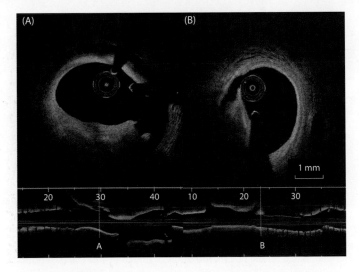

Figure 4.13 **Dissections that should be shielded.** (A) Long dissection with a larger flap dimension. (B) Dissection of lipid-rich plaque.

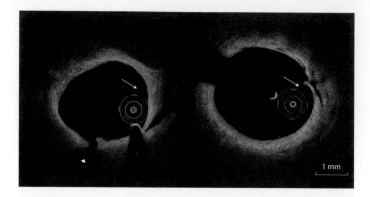

Figure 4.14 Smaller thin dissections (white arrows) can be left without additional stenting. The arrowhead on the left panel indicates a side branch.

4.4.5 Incomplete lesion coverage

Geographic miss might occur if one does not carefully perform preprocedure OCT lesion assessment to compare or coregister with angiography. Since higher residual plaque volume, particularly necrotic core-rich plaque at the stent edge, is known to be associated with target lesion failure,[18] careful reading of OCT pullback image and stent planning is needed. Geographic miss should be suspected when you find stent edges located on a large amount of plaque and/or lipid-rich attenuated plaque where the OCT signal cannot penetrate (Figure 4.15). Since the calculation of residual plaque burden is not feasible by OCT,

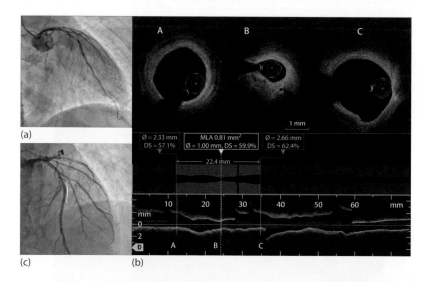

Figure 4.15 Case 5. Geographic miss due to inappropriate stent selection. Target lesion was 90% stenosis in the proximal left anterior descending artery (a). Based on the preprocedural OCT lumen profile (b), the optimal stent length should have been about 24 mm. Without utilizing this OCT finding, the operator selected a 2.75 × 18 mm Xience Xpedition (c, white line indicates the stented segment). *(Continued)*

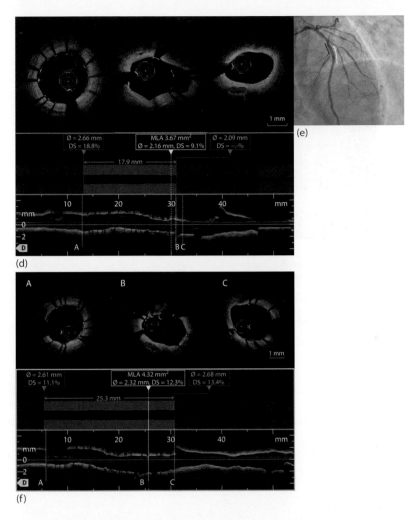

Figure 4.15 (Continued) Case 5. Geographic miss due to inappropriate stent selection. Despite the favorable appearance of the angiogram, the stent was deployed on the thin-cap fibroatheroma at the proximal edge of the OCT image (d). Therefore, another 3.0 × 12 mm Xience Xpedition was deployed, overlapped with the first stent, followed by postdilation ([e] black line indicates the segment deployed with the second stent). On final OCT, the thin-cap fibroatheroma was fully sealed (f).

the necessity of additional stenting must be judged comprehensively, considering plaque type (lipid-rich plaque) and residual minimal lumen area, for that IVUS cutoff value is different between the proximal and distal edges.[19]

4.4.6 Tissue prolapse

OCT is useful for evaluating tissue prolapse after stenting (Figure 4.16). Compared with IVUS, OCT detects tissue prolapse between stent struts with more sensitivity.[20,21] Tissue prolapse was not associated with clinical outcomes during hospitalization and at late follow-up,[22,23] while post-PCI myocardial injury was related to

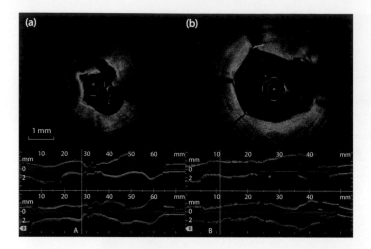

Figure 4.16 Large plaque protrusion in the deployed stent. Corresponding OCT images of preprocedure (a) and poststenting (b). At the site of minimal lumen area (MLA), a thin cap of ruptured plaque was observed preprocedure.

the volume of prolapsed tissue.[23] As long as the achieved minimal stent area is acceptable, additional post–balloon inflation at the site of tissue prolapse seems to be unnecessary.

4.5   CONCLUSION

Various OCT applications for optimal stent deployment, including vessel preparation, stent planning, and stent assessment, have been widely recognized following the introduction of frequency-domain OCT. Making good use of OCT can yield better procedural outcomes that are strongly associated with improved clinical outcomes.

REFERENCES

1. Nakamura S et al. Intracoronary ultrasound observations during stent implantation. *Circulation* 1994;89:2026–34.
2. Görge G et al. Intravascular ultrasound after low and high inflation pressure coronary artery stent implantation. *Journal of the American College of Cardiology* 1995;26:725–30.
3. Mudra H et al. Ultrasound guidance of Palmaz-Schatz intracoronary stenting with a combined intravascular ultrasound balloon catheter. *Circulation* 1994;90:1252–61.
4. Brodie BR et al. Is adjunctive balloon postdilatation necessary after coronary stent deployment? Final results from the POSTIT trial. *Catheter and Cardiovascular Interventions* 2003;59:184–92.
5. Kumbhani DJ et al. Role of aspiration and mechanical thrombectomy in patients with acute myocardial infarction undergoing primary angioplasty: An updated meta-analysis of randomized trials. *Journal of the American College of Cardiology* 2013;62:1409–18.
6. Attizzani GF et al. Mechanisms, pathophysiology, and clinical aspects of incomplete stent apposition. *Journal of the American College of Cardiology* 2014;63:1355–67.
7. Kajander OA et al. Feasibility and repeatability of optical coherence tomography measurements of pre-stent thrombus burden in patients with STEMI treated with primary PCI. *European Heart Journal Cardiovascular Imaging* 2015;16:96–107.
8. Prati F et al. OCT-based diagnosis and management of STEMI associated with intact fibrous cap. *JACC Cardiovascular Imaging* 2013;6:283–7.

9. Prati F et al. Angiography alone versus angiography plus optical coherence tomography to guide decision-making during percutaneous coronary intervention: The Centro per la Lotta contro l'Infarto-Optimisation of Percutaneous Coronary Intervention (CLI-OPCI) study. *EuroIntervention* 2012;8:823–9.

10. Imola F et al. Association between proximal stent edge positioning on atherosclerotic plaques containing lipid pools and postprocedural myocardial infarction (from the CLI-POOL Study). *American Journal of Cardiology* 2013;4:526–31.

11. Fujino Y et al. Impact of main-branch calcified plaque on side-branch stenosis in bifurcation stenting: An optical coherence tomography study. *International Journal of Cardiology* 2014;176:1056–60.

12. Cook S et al. Incomplete stent apposition and very late stent thrombosis after drug-eluting stent implantation. *Circulation* 2007;115:2426–34.

13. Windecker S, Meier B. Late coronary stent thrombosis. *Circulation* 2007;116:1952–65.

14. Fujii K et al. Stent underexpansion and residual reference segment stenosis are related to stent thrombosis after sirolimus-eluting stent implantation: An intravascular ultrasound study. *Journal of the American College of Cardiology* 2005;45:995–8.

15. Inoue T et al. Impact of strut-vessel distance and underlying plaque type on the resolution of acute strut malapposition: Serial optimal coherence tomography analysis after everolimus-eluting stent implantation. *International Journal of Cardiovascular Imaging* 2014;30:857–65.

16. Alegría-Barrero E et al. Optical coherence tomography for guidance of distal cell recrossing in bifurcation stenting: Choosing the right cell matters. *EuroIntervention* 2012;8:205–13.

17. Chamié D et al. Incidence, predictors, morphological characteristics, and clinical outcomes of stent edge dissections detected by optical coherence tomography. *JACC Cardiovascular Interventions* 2013;6:800–13.

18. Gogas BD et al. Edge vascular response after percutaneous coronary intervention: An intracoronary ultrasound and optical coherence tomography appraisal: From radioactive platforms to first- and second-generation drug-eluting stents and bioresorbable scaffolds. *JACC Cardiovascular Interventions* 2013;6:211–21.

19. Kang SJ et al. Intravascular ultrasound predictors for edge restenosis after newer generation drug-eluting stent implantation. *American Journal of Cardiology* 2013;111:1408–14.

20. Sohn J et al. A comparison of tissue prolapse with optical coherence tomography and intravascular ultrasound after drug-eluting stent implantation. *International Journal of Cardiovascular Imaging* 2015;31:21–2.

21. Bezerra HG et al. Optical coherence tomography versus intravascular ultrasound to evaluate coronary artery disease and percutaneous coronary intervention. *JACC Cardiovascular Interventions* 2013;6:228–36.

22. Jin QH et al. Incidence, predictors, and clinical impact of tissue prolapse after coronary intervention: An intravascular optical coherence tomography study. *Cardiology* 2011;119:197–203.

23. Sugiyama T et al. Quantitative assessment of tissue prolapse on optical coherence tomography and its relation to underlying plaque morphologies and clinical outcome in patients with elective stent implantation. *International Journal of Cardiology* 2014;176:182–90.

Chapter 5

OCT for left main assessment

Yusuke Fujino

5.1 INTRODUCTION

Percutaneous coronary intervention (PCI) of unprotected left main (ULM) coronary artery disease has gained significant adoption over the past decade.[1,2] This mode of therapy, however, demands high procedural precision, given the large amount of myocardium at risk, and it is often difficult to assess the dimensions of ULM. The efficacy of intravascular ultrasound (IVUS) systems during PCI was reported previously[3,4] and has made significant contributions to our current understanding and treatment of ULM disease.[5] The role of optical coherence tomography (OCT) guiding PCI has been recently demonstrated by our group and others.[6–8] In this scenario, the possibility of imaging the ULM using OCT is attractive. However, the first-generation time-domain OCT systems had a relatively narrow field of view and required proximal vessel occlusion for image acquisition, precluding its application in ULM. Conversely, frequency-domain optical coherence tomography (FD-OCT) technology allows pullback speeds up to 25 mm/s, which obviates the need for proximal vessel occlusion. FD-OCT also offers a larger (10 mm) field of view, enabling visualization of large vessels, such as the ULM.

In this section, we evaluate the safety and feasibility of FD-OCT for ULM disease based on our data and representative cases.

5.2 SAFETY OF FD-OCT FOR ULM DISEASE

The safety of FD-OCT during non-ULM PCI was reported increasingly; however, there are no data evaluating the safety during ULM PCI. Regarding the safety of FD-OCT, we compared it with that of IVUS, which has been established safe for ULM PCI. We prospectively evaluated 35 patients who underwent ULM PCI with both modalities.[9] In this study, we evaluated the coronary artery stent thrombosis (ST) changes, dissections, arrhythmias, slow flow, and spasms pre-PCI (before ballooning, stent implantation, and any device interaction) and post-PCI. Table 5.1 shows the angiographic characteristics of these patients. In order to acquire the clear OCT image, we usually need to inject a relatively large amount of contrast and velocity for ULM because of the large vessel size. In spite of the large amount and velocity of injected contrast, there were no severe complications in modality during both pre-PCI and post-PCI, except one case presenting an ST change because of a tight stenosis lesion (Table 5.2). FD-OCT was performed safely during pre-PCI and post-PCI of ULM PCI.

TABLE 5.1
Angiographic characteristics (n = 35)

Lesion location	n (%)
Ostial only, n (%)	0 (0)
Midshaft only, n (%)	1 (2.9)
Distal only, n (%)	22 (62.9)
Ostial and midshaft, n (%)	0 (0)
Midshaft and distal, n (%)	11 (31.4)
Ostial and distal, n (%)	1 (2.9)
Ostial and midshaft distal, n (%)	0 (0)
Medina classification	n (%)
(1,1,1), n (%)	7 (20)
(1,1,0), n (%)	9 (25.7)
(1,0,1), n (%)	1 (2.9)
(1,0,0), n (%)	3 (8.6)
(0,1,1), n (%)	5 (14.3)
(0,1,0), n (%)	9 (25.7)
(0,0,1), n (%)	1 (2.9)
QCA	n (%)
Nonstented segment	
MLD (mm)	0.96 ± 0.37
RVD (mm)	3.5 ± 0.70
%DS	72.6 ± 8.6
Stented segment	
MLD (mm)	3.14 ± 0.53
RVD (mm)	3.54 ± 0.53
%DS	9.03 ± 4.00

Note: %DS, percentage diameter stenosis; MLD, minimum lumen diameter; QCA, quantitative coronary analysis; RVD, reference vessel diameter.

TABLE 5.2
Imagine procedure characteristics ($n = 35$)

	IVUS	FD-OCT	*p* value
Pre-PCI			
Safety			
ST change	1 (2.9)	1 (2.9)	1
Dissection	0 (0.0)	0 (0.0)	N/A
Arrhythmia	0 (0.0)	0 (0.0)	N/A
Slow flow	0 (0.0)	0 (0.0)	N/A
Volume of contrast			
Total volume of contract dye/pullback (mL)	0	17.8 ± 6.2	N/A
Velocity rate (mL/s)	0	4.7 ± 0.56	N/A
Post-PCI			
Safety			
ST change	0 (0.0)	0 (0.0)	N/A
Dissection	0 (0.0)	0 (0.0)	N/A
Arrhythmia	0 (0.0)	0 (0.0)	N/A
Slow flow	0 (0.0)	0 (0.0)	N/A
Spasm	0 (0.0)	0 (0.0)	N/A
Volume of contrast			
Total volume of contract dye/pullback (mL)	0	18.7 ± 6.7	N/A
Velocity rate (mL/s)	0	4.9 ± 0.57	N/A

Note: N/A, not applicable.

5.3   FD-OCT MEASUREMENTS FOR ULM DISEASE

Great advantage of FD-OCT for ULM was the larger field of view compared with the first-generation time-domain OCT systems. FD-OCT offers a larger (10 mm) field of view, enabling visualization of large vessels, such as the left main coronary artery (LMCA).[6] Because of the high-resolution image, FD-OCT can provide clear intracoronary structures, such as coronary dissection, malapposed stent struts, and thrombosis.

Before discussing the feasibility of FD-OCT for ULM, we present the data showing measurement of the lumen, the stent area, detection of malapposition, the thrombus, and edge dissection, compared with IVUS.

As Table 5.3 shows, FD-OCT measurements for ULM lesion were acceptable compared with those of IVUS, as well as for non-ULM lesion, which was reported previously. The lumen and stent area were comparable between FD-OCT and IVUS, and in most of the cases, FD-OCT could provide a whole cross-sectional image without being out of screen. In particular, the detection of tissue protruding, malapposition, and distal edge dissection were much higher in FD-OCT. Based on these results, FD-OCT measurements of ULM lesion were reliable during PCI compared with IVUS.

TABLE 5.3
IVUS and FD-OCT imaging analysis (n = 35)

	IVUS	FD-OCT	p value
Pre-PCI			
Lumen area (mm^2)			
Mean	7.58 ± 2.61	7.60 ± 2.63	0.936
Minimum	3.46 ± 1.66	2.94 ± 1.77	0.002
Intraluminal thrombus, n (%)	0 (0.00)	3 (9.4)	0.081
Vessel out of screen, n (%)	N/A	1 (0.1)	N/A
Post-PCI			
Lumen area (mm^2)			
Mean	10.85 ± 2.47	11.24 ± 2.66	0.132
Minimum 7.21 ± 2.23	7.18 ± 2.15	0.875	0.875
Stent area (mm^2)			
Mean	10.44 ± 2.33	10.49 ± 2.32	0.821
Minimum	6.88 ± 2.03	6.79 ± 2.09	0.534
Tissue protruding area (mm^2)	0.11 ± 0.07	0.23 ± 0.09	<0.001
Malapposition area (mm^2)	0.12 ± 0.36	0.43 ± 0.51	<0.001
Malapposition volume (mm^2)	1.95 ± 5.69	7.73 ± 7.60	<0.001
Intraluminal thrombus, n (%)	0 (0.00)	2 (5.9)	0.154
Proximal edge dissection, n (%)	0 (0.00)	1 (3.0)	0.317
Distal edge dissection, n (%)	2 (6.1)	10 (30.3)	0.011

Note: N/A, not applicable.

5.4   FEASIBILITY OF FD-OCT FOR ULM DISEASE

In this section, we show the representative cases, which show the feasibility of FD-OCT for detecting the PCI strategy.

A patient who presented with chest pain with elevated cardiac enzyme underwent emergent coronary angiogram. Figure 5.1a shows the coronary angiogram. Coronary angiogram could not detect the culprit lesion clearly; however, FD-OCT clearly showed the huge amount of red thrombus in the distal LMCA (Figure 5.1b).

Figure 5.2a and b shows angiograms of patients with a history of hemodialysis who underwent stent implantation from LMCA to the left anterior descendent artery (LAD). In this case, we could see the coronary dissection behind the calcified plaque of the LMCA body using FD-OCT, which is not clear in IVUS (Figure 5.2c), and implanted an additional stent.

Patients who underwent everolimus-eluting stent (EES) implantation from the LMCA to the LAD and FD-OCT showed obvious malapposed stent struts in the LMCA body (Figure 5.3a). Based on this image, we added additional balloon angioplasty and acquired good stent apposition (Figure 5.3b).

Furthermore, FD-OCT can show clear stent strut, especially in the bifurcation lesion. The next case shows an LMCA patient who underwent kissing balloon inflation (KBT) after stent implantation from the LMCA body to the LAD. Before KBT, the FD-OCT showed jailed stent struts in the left circumflex artery (LCX) ostium (Figure 5.4a). After KBT to the LMCA-LAD/LCX, FD-OCT showed the apposed stent

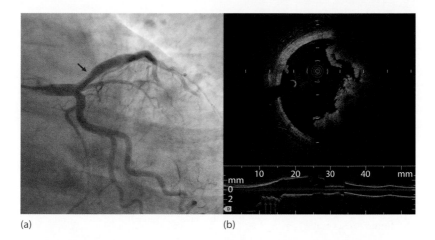

(a)   (b)

Figure 5.1 (a) Patients with chest pain and elevated cardiac enzyme underwent emergent coronary angiogram, which showed a radiolucent lesion of the proximal LAD (red arrow). (b) FD-OCT clearly shows the red thrombus in the proximal LAD in a cross section and longitudinal image (red arrows).

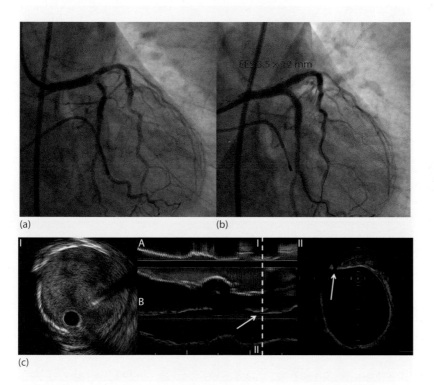

Figure 5.2 (a and b) Coronary angiogram shows a lesion with severe calcified plaque of the proximal LAD, and EES (3.5 × 12 mm) implantation was performed. (c) FD-OCT and IVUS were performed from the LMCA-LAD. Proximal stent edge dissections were identified by FD-OCT but unrevealed by IVUS. Panel I: (A) An IVUS longitudinal view of a stented segment. The cross-sectional image corresponding to the white dashed line is represented in (I); no pathological findings are demonstrated. The corresponding FD-OCT longitudinal view showing a dissection in the proximal edge of the stent is revealed in B (white arrow). Panel II: The coregistered cross-sectional image demonstrates an edge dissection in a calcified plaque (white arrow).

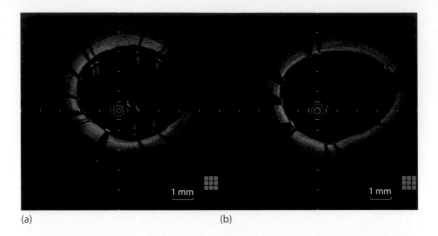

(a)   (b)

Figure 5.3 (a) FD-OCT shows the clear malapposed stent struts (red arrows) after EES (3.5 × 23 mm) implantation of the LMCA body. (b) An additional noncompliance balloon (4.5 × 10 mm) was inflated, and well-apposed stent struts are shown by FD-OCT.

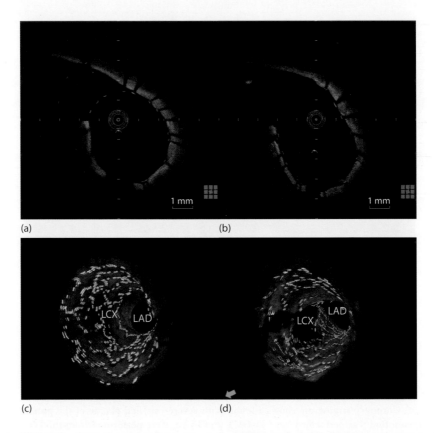

(a)   (b)

(c)   (d)

Figure 5.4 (a) An EES (3.5 × 23 mm) was implanted from the LMCA to the LAD. Malapposed stent struts are shown in the LCX ostium. (b) After KBT (LMCA-LAD 3.5 × 23 mm)/LMCA-LCX 3.0 × 15 mm), stent struts were attached to the LCX ostium and well-apposed stent struts apposition were shown by FD-OCT. (c) 3D reconstruction image of LMCA bifurcation before KBT. Jailed stent struts were clearly sown in the LCX ostium. (d) 3D reconstruction image of LMCA bifurcation after KBT. There were no jailed stent struts of the LCX ostium after KBT.

struts of the LCX ostium (Figure 5.4b). Additionally, using three-dimensional (3D) reconstructed software, 3D reconstructed images can show the very clear stent apposition comparing before KBT and after KBT (Figure 5.4c and d).

FD-OCT can also correct the procedure mistake that is caused by geographic miss by the coronary angiogram. Figure 5.5a shows a case where the patient underwent a KBT procedure after stent implantation from the LMCA to the LAD. The angiogram shows successful KBT (Figure 5.5b); however, FD-OCT clearly shows a residual stent strut of the LCX ostium (Figure 5.5c and d). Sometimes PCI is undergone with only coronary angiogram; however, for this case the coronary angiogram involves a geographic miss. FD-OCT has the potential to correct the geographic miss, which is not shown in the coronary angiogram.

Anatomically, the vessel size of the LMCA is relatively large compared with the size of the non-LMCA vessel.

Because of the large vessel size, sometimes we need to pay attention to stent apposition against vessel wall and the guidewire position. Figure 5.6a shows a case with a lesion just proximal to the LAD; the patient underwent stent implantation from the LMCA to the LAD following KBT to LMCA-LAD/LCX (Figure 5.6b). Figure 5.6c shows a good angiogram after KBT; however, FD-OCT images show (Figure 5.6d) that there were malapposed stent struts in the LMCA body. In this case, at first the guidewire crossed out of

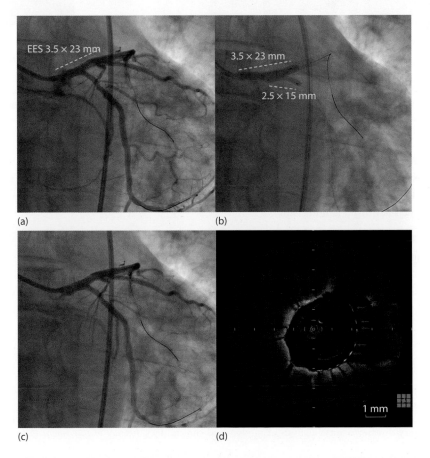

(a)　　　　　　　　　　　(b)

(c)　　　　　　　　　　　(d)

Figure 5.5 (a) An EES (3.5 × 23 mm) was implanted from the LMCA to the LAD. (b) KBT (LMCA-LAD 3.5 × 23 mm/ LMCA-LCX 2.5 × 15 mm) was performed. Coronary angiogram shows a successful KBT result. (c) Successful KBT is shown in the coronary angiogram; however, FD-OCT shows the malapposed stent struts (red arrows) of the LCX ostium (d).

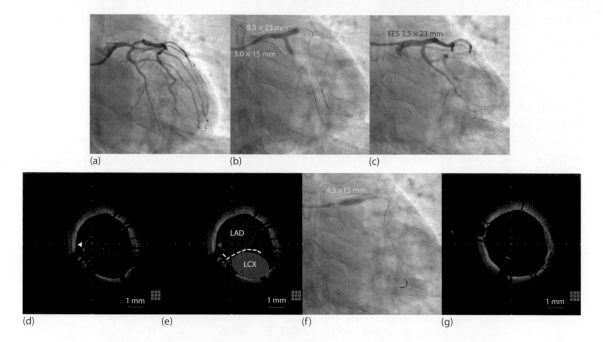

Figure 5.6 (a) Angiogram shows a narrowing in distal unprotected left main coronary artery (ULMCA)/origin of the LAD. (b) EES implantation (3.5 × 23 mm) from the ULMCA to the LAD following KBT (LMCA-LAD 3.5 × 23 mm/ LMCA-LCX 3.0 × 15 mm). (c) Favorable angiogram after KBT; however, (d and e) FD-OCT shows the malapposed stent struts (red arrows) between the guidewire of the LAD (white arrowhead) and the LCX (red arrowhead). After balloon angioplasty (noncompliance balloon 4.5 × 15 mm) of the LMCA (f), FD-OCT shows the well-apposed stent struts (g).

the stent struts at the LMCA ostium, and then the guidewire crossed into the inside of the stent and into the LCX. During KBT, the LAD and LCX balloon were inflated between the implanted stent (Figure 5.6e). Based on the FD-OCT image, additional balloon angioplasty (Figure 5.6g) was performed and apposed stent apposition was acquired (Figure 5.6f).

5.5 CONCLUSIONS

FD-OCT assessment during ULM PCI was safe and feasible. Further studies are necessary to evaluate the impact of OCT for ULM PCI on the clinical outcomes.

REFERENCES

1. Mehilli J et al. Paclitaxel- versus sirolimus-eluting stents for unprotected left main coronary artery disease. *Journal of the American College of Cardiology* 2009;53:1760–8.
2. Capodanno D et al. Percutaneous coronary intervention versus coronary artery bypass graft surgery in left main coronary artery disease: A meta-analysis of randomized clinical data. *Journal of the American College of Cardiology* 2011;58:1426–32.
3. Fitzgerald PJ et al. Final results of the Can Routine Ultrasound Influence Stent Expansion (CRUISE) study. *Circulation* 2000;5:523–30.

4. Oemrawsingh PV et al. Intravascular ultrasound guidance improves angiographic and clinical outcome of stent implantation for long coronary artery stenoses: Final results of a randomized comparison with angiographic guidance (TULIP Study). *Circulation* 2003;1:62–7.

5. Park SJ et al. Impact of intravascular ultrasound guidance on long-term mortality in stenting for unprotected left main coronary artery stenosis. *Circulation Cardiovascular Interventions* 2009;2:167–77.

6. Stefano G et al. Unrestricted utilization of frequency domain optical coherence tomography in coronary interventions. *International Journal of Cardiovascular Imaging* 2013;4:741–52.

7. Yoon JH et al. Feasibility and safety of the second-generation, frequency domain optical coherence tomography (FD-OCT): A multicenter study. *Journal of Invasive Cardiology* 2012;24:206–9.

8. Prati F et al. Angiography alone versus angiography plus optical coherence tomography to guide decision-making during percutaneous coronary intervention: The Centro per la Lotta contro l'Infarto-Optimisation of Percutaneous Coronary Intervention (CLI-OPCI) study. *EuroIntervention* 2012;7:823–9.

9. Fujino Y et al. Frequency-domain optical coherence tomography assessment of unprotected left main coronary artery disease—A comparison with intravascular ultrasound. *Catheterization and Cardiovascular Intervention* 2013;3:173–83.

Chapter 6

Optical coherence tomography for late stent failure

Tej Sheth, Anthony Fung, and Catalin Toma

6.1 INTRODUCTION

Although coronary stent technology continues to improve over time, clinical events from previously placed stents are commonly encountered. The two principal modes of late stent failure are in-stent restenosis and late stent thrombosis (ST). In both cases, a mechanistic understanding of the causes of stent failure may be obtained with optical coherence tomography (OCT). The excellent near-field resolution of OCT and the clear delineation of the stent vessel interface allow for the evaluation of intracoronary stents in great detail. Patients with stent failure are at elevated risk for recurrent events. OCT-based management has the potential to improve acute and long-term results in these patients.

6.2 RESTENOSIS

6.2.1 Pathobiology of restenosis

Early healing responses following stent implantation involve the deposition of fibrin, migration of inflammatory cells, and initiation of endothelialization. Subsequently, smooth muscle proliferation and extracellular matrix synthesis lead to the development of a neointima rich in collagen and proteoglycans. The smooth muscle cells and collagen fibers give normal neointima optical signals that are similar to those of fibrous tissue. Neointimal proliferation is the main cause of stent restenosis within the first 2 years of implantation.[1] Beyond this period, further progression of neointima usually involves development of neoatherosclerosis. Pathologic analyses demonstrate a time-dependent development of various atherosclerotic changes inside stented segments, including the formation of fibroatheroma, which may become thin capped and can rupture, while calcification was less frequent.[2]

6.2.2 OCT patterns of restenosis

Angiographic patterns of restenosis have been described previously as focal, diffuse, stent edge, and occlusive.[3] OCT provides complementary understanding of the distribution of restenosis in the stent, as well as insight into the composition of the neointima. Three principle morphologic patterns of the neointima have been identified on OCT (Figure 6.1). Homogenous neointima has high-backscattering and low-attenuation characteristics due to the high content of smooth muscle cells and collagen fibers.[4] Homogeneous neointima is the appearance of the normal in-stent proliferative response. In addition to homogenous neointima, OCT can demonstrate layered and heterogeneous healing patterns. Layered neointima has a high-backscattering superficial layer and a deeper layer with low-backscattering properties. Heterogenous neointima has a speckled pattern with areas of high and low backscattering distributed throughout the tissue.[5] Although low-backscattering areas of the neointima have not been well characterized histologically, fibrin accumulation, organized thrombus, and inflammation can produce this appearance on OCT.[4] In practice, several different patterns of neointimal tissue in different regions of the same stent are frequently encountered.

Prospective data suggest that patterns of neointima may differ in their rates of stent-related clinical outcomes. With image characterization performed at 8–9 months postimplant and a median follow-up of 31 months, heterogeneous neointima was associated with a 13.7% rate of adverse cardiac events compared with 7.3% for layered and 2.9% for homogenous.[5] These findings suggest that heterogenous neointima may be more likely to progress. It may perhaps share some features with the early stages of neoatherosclerosis.[6]

OCT findings indicating neoatherosclerosis include the presence of lipid-rich plaques, thin-cap fibroatheroma, plaque rupture, and calcification (Figure 6.2). In bare-metal stents, the prevalence of neoatherosclerotic changes increases with increasing duration from implant and appears to be accompanied by increased neovascularization.[7] In drug-eluting stents (DESs), neoatherosclerotic changes are seen earlier[8] and progressively increase over time.[9] It is unclear which components of DES technology (drug or polymer) contribute to this phenomenon, and relatively few patients with second-generation DESs have been studied.

Increased stent age, use of DESs, and vascular risk factors are associated with the presence of neoatherosclerosis on OCT examination.[10] Neoatherosclerosis appears to contribute to many cases of late stent failure. In one series of patients undergoing late clinically driven target lesion revascularization (TLR), the incidence

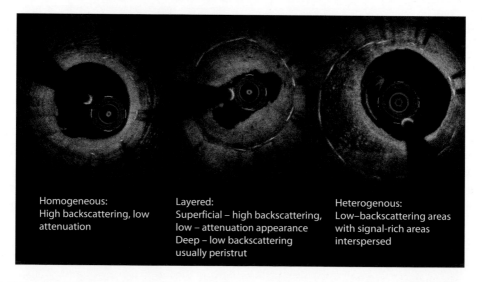

Figure 6.1 Types of neointima.

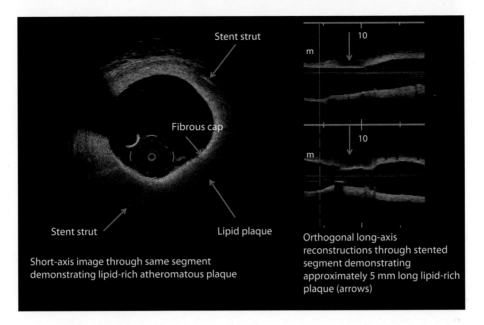

Figure 6.2 Lipid-rich in-stent plaque.

of in-stent lipid-rich neointima was 100%, and that of both thin-cap fibroatheroma and plaque rupture was >50%, suggesting that in-stent neoatherosclerosis with plaque rupture is a common cause of late bare-metal[11] and DES restenosis.[9]

6.2.3 Management

OCT-guided management of restenosis includes several components. The OCT images can be evaluated to determine the spatial distribution of the restenosis. In the DES era, restenosis is often due to mechanical factors and may be present predominantly at the stent margins (Figure 6.3). Figure 6.3 illustrates moderate eccentric in-stent neointimal proliferation in a Taxus stent with a very severe distal edge proliferative response. Geographic miss during the original PCI is the suspected etiology. Note the minimal late lumen loss in the stented segment.

An additional mechanical feature that can contribute to restenosis is chronic stent underexpansion. The in-stent cross-sectional area can be readily measured and compared at different points throughout the stent by OCT. Figure 6.4 demonstrates chronic stent underexpansion that contributed to bare-metal stent failure at 6 months after implant. The minimum stent area was in the middle of the stented segment at the point of overlap between two stents. The stent area at this point was 4.21 mm², compared with 6.73 mm² distally and 5.80 mm² proximally. This segment was expanded with noncompliant balloon inflation prior to additional device treatment. Follow-up OCT showed that the stent area was expanded to 6.2 mm² (Figure 6.4).

In restenosis cases, initial lesion preparation usually involves predilatation with compliant or noncompliant balloons. OCT can help to identify appropriate balloon length and position to avoid reinjury of well-healed portions of the neointima. Figure 6.5 shows the tissue response to balloon inflation with a cutting balloon. The first angiogram and OCT are taken after dilatation with compliant 2.0 mm and noncompliant 2.75 mm balloons, revealing significant residual neointimal tissue. After dilatation with a 3.0 × 10 mm cutting balloon, satisfactory debulking is achieved with a "stent-like" result (Figure 6.5).

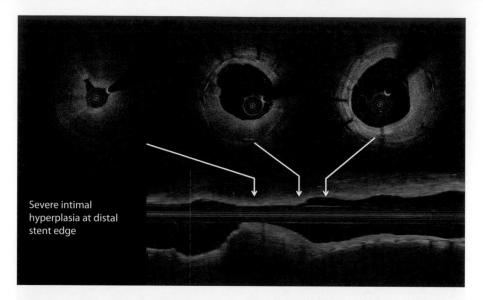

Severe intimal hyperplasia at distal stent edge

Figure 6.3 Distal edge restenosis.

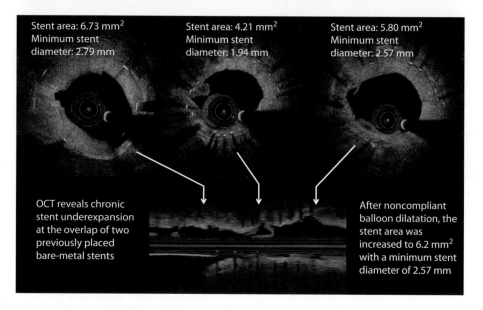

Stent area: 6.73 mm^2
Minimum stent diameter: 2.79 mm

Stent area: 4.21 mm^2
Minimum stent diameter: 1.94 mm

Stent area: 5.80 mm^2
Minimum stent diameter: 2.57 mm

OCT reveals chronic stent underexpansion at the overlap of two previously placed bare-metal stents

After noncompliant balloon dilatation, the stent area was increased to 6.2 mm^2 with a minimum stent diameter of 2.57 mm

Figure 6.4 Stent underexpansion.

Once adequate lesion preparation has been performed, options for further treatments include the use of drug-eluting balloons (DEBs) or implantation of additional stents. Comparative trials suggest that DEBs and DESs have similar clinical efficacies for the treatment of bare-metal and DES restenosis.[12,13] The choice between the two strategies may be influenced by operator preference and clinical factors. OCT factors that may favor DEB include (1) persistent stent underexpansion that cannot be satisfactorily resolved with balloon dilatation, (2) substantial areas of lack of coverage of the initial stent,[14] (3) the presence of a major side branch, (4) multiple layers of prior stent implants, and (5) small stent diameter. OCT factors that may favor DESs include (1) extensive intrastent tissue, particularly with neoatherosclerotic characteristics; (2) the presence of a

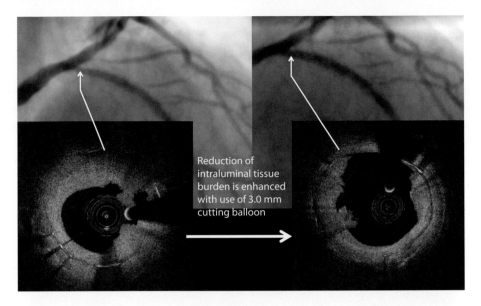

Reduction of intraluminal tissue burden is enhanced with use of 3.0 mm cutting balloon

Figure 6.5 Cutting balloon debulking.

prior stent that is well expanded and deeply embedded in the vessel wall; (3) nonuniform stent strut distribution due to placement of the stent in a highly angulated segment; and (4) the inability to achieve a stent-like result with balloon dilatation.

6.3 CASE REPORT: IN-STENT RESTENOSIS

A 45-year-old female insulin-requiring diabetes patient presented with recurrent Canadian Cardiovascular Society (CCS) III angina. She underwent left anterior descendent artery (LAD) bare-metal stent implantation 5 years prior. She developed recurrent angina 2 years ago. The LAD stent was patent, but there was a new total occlusion of the left circumflex artery (LCX). This was treated with implantation of two bare-metal stents. One year later, she represented with angina. Angiography demonstrated continued patency of her LAD stent and severe restenosis in the mid-LCX just beyond the first obtuse marginal branch (Figure 6.6). This lesion was treated with two everolimus-eluting stents (Promus 2.5 × 12 mm and 2.75 × 12 mm).

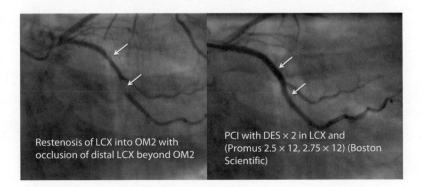

Restenosis of LCX into OM2 with occlusion of distal LCX beyond OM2

PCI with DES × 2 in LCX and (Promus 2.5 × 12, 2.75 × 12) (Boston Scientific)

Figure 6.6 Bare-metal restenosis treated with a DES.

After 1 year, symptoms recurred, progressing to CCS IV angina. Angiography showed restenosis of the LCX with thrombolysis in myocardial infarction (TIMI) 2 flow. Predilatation was performed with a 2 mm balloon (Figure 6.7). Once flow was restored, OCT imaging was carried out (Figure 6.8). The existing stents were well expanded with a stent area of 6.38 mm^2 at the distal segment, 7.36 mm^2 at the midbody, and 6.65 mm^2 at the proximal segment. Different healing patterns were seen. The appearance was predominantly homogenous at the level of the OM1 branch and distally. In the proximal stent, the appearance was layered with circumferential peristrut low-backscattering tissue. Due to multiple layers of prior stenting and the desire to avoid rejailing the OM1 branch, the lesion was treated with DEBs. After excluding the well-healed distal stented segment, two 15 mm treatment zones were identified on either side of the OM branch (Figure 6.9) for retreatment. Both of these arterial segments were treated with 3.0 × 15 mm Pantera Lux (Biotronik) DEBs. Final OCT imaging (Figure 6.10) demonstrates that there is minimal residual intrastent tissue and significant enlargement of the lumen.

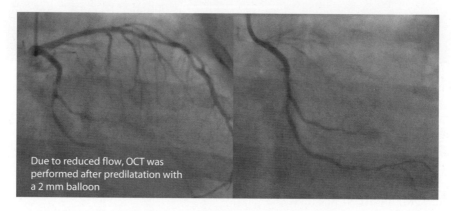

Figure 6.7 Repeat restenosis treated with a percutaneous balloon angioplasty (PTCA) balloon prior to OCT imaging.

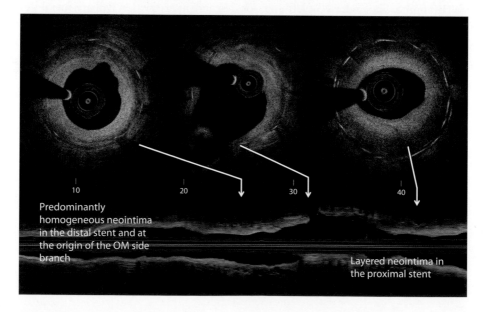

Figure 6.8 OCT imaging following predilatation.

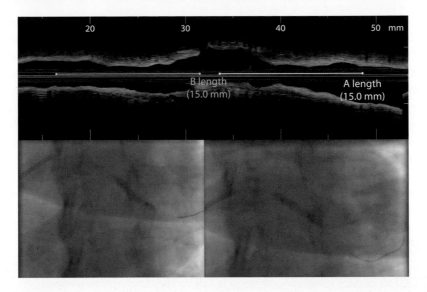

Figure 6.9 Treatment with a DEB.

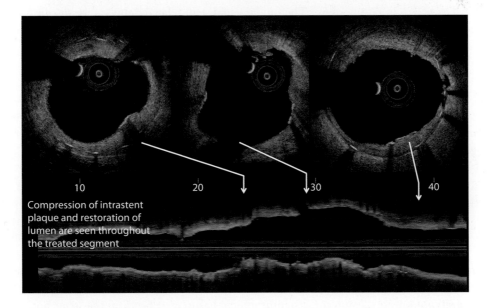

Figure 6.10 OCT imaging following DEB treatment.

6.4   STENT THROMBOSIS

6.4.1   Prevalence and etiology of stent thrombosis

Acute thrombus formation inside a coronary stent generally presents as ST-elevation myocardial infarction (STEMI) with significant associated morbidity and mortality.[15] Although the incidence of ST has decreased with second-generation stent platforms and novel antiplatelet agents, given the large number of patients treated with coronary stents in the past decades, this complication continues to be problematic. At one of our institutions (University of Pittsburgh Medical Center), the observed rate of STEMI resulting from late or very late ST in 2012–2013 was 8.0%, comparable to the findings of Brodie et al.[16] showing an increasing frequency of ST over time among STEMI patients (6.0% in 2003–2004 to 10.9% in 2009–2010). Although more frequent with first-generation DESs, it is important to note that these events are also seen with newer-generation DESs, as well as bare-metal stents.

ST can be classified based on timing from implantation as acute (<1 day), subacute (1–30 days), late (30 days to 1 year), and very late (>1 year). The causal events leading to ST are often multifactorial, with several mechanisms interacting to create a perfect-storm scenario. This may include patient-related factors, medication compliance issues, inflammatory states associated with surgical procedures or malignancy, and the underlying intrastent pathology. While the causality and pathology for acute or subacute ST is often easy to identify (i.e., mechanical or medication-related issues), this is less so for late or very late ST. In contemporary practice, two-thirds of ST occurs late after implantation.[17] In the DESERT study, the majority of ST events occurred after 1 year following implant (75%) and, importantly, continued to occur for the duration of the study (up to 7.3 years of follow-up).[18]

6.4.2   Role of OCT to identify intrastent pathology in late or very late stent thrombosis

The pathologic mechanism of late ST has been studied *in vivo* with intravascular ultrasound (IVUS) or OCT,[19] as well as *ex vivo* in postmortem.[2] The fundamental stent-related nidus can be distilled down to two broad categories, namely, lack of tissue coverage on the stent struts[19] and intrastent neoatherosclerosis.[20]

Incomplete tissue coverage can be found in three different scenarios, depending on the position of the stent struts relative to the vessel wall.

1. *Lack of stent endothelialization*: A scenario seen earlier postimplant is that of a well-expanded and apposed stent, with thrombus originating on struts with no tissue coverage. This delayed reendothelialization is the adverse consequence of the antimitotic drugs.[21] Although the OCT does not have adequate resolution to image a single layer of endothelial cells, struts with limited tissue coverage are relatively easy to identify as having virtually no neointima on top and being bright with sharp margins. A good example of uncovered struts is seen when performing OCT immediately following stent implantation. Uncovered stent struts are commonly seen with early ST presentation (<30 days) following premature discontinuation of dual antiplatelet therapy, but are relatively rarely seen with late stent thrombosis in second-generation DESs due to the improved reendothelialization with these devices.

2. *Persistent malapposition*: A scenario where the stent is not apposed sufficiently at the time of the original procedure, and this can serve as a nidus for thrombus formation later on. For the strut malapposition to persist long-term, a significant gap has to exist between the struts and the vessel wall (usually >300 microns), with smaller degrees of malapposition resolving over time.[22] OCT reveals a blood-filled space behind the stent struts, with thrombus present at the site of malapposition, often with extension behind the struts as well.

3. *Acquired malapposition*: A different mechanism of malapposition that occurs late in a stent that was initially well expanded and apposed. In cases of acute coronary syndrome, resolution of the thrombus trapped behind the stent can lead to a gap between the struts and the vessel wall later on. A separate mechanism specific to DESs is that of positive vessel remodeling, where outward aneurysmal dilatation occurs as a reaction to the cytotoxic drugs or hypersensitivity response to the polymer. The term *coronary evagination* is used to describe these fingerlike limited aneurysms.[23] We find

that three-dimensional OCT can be useful in this scenario, revealing a typical pitted appearance of the vessel wall with divots inside the stent cells. The stent struts are sometimes devoid of tissue coverage in this case, and adherent thrombus can be easily identified. Unlike the persistent malapposition described above, the vessel diameter at the site of the acquired malapposition is larger than the vessel diameter of the proximal or distal reference segments. Examination of the OCT images in the longitudinal view is useful in understanding the contour of the stent relative to the vessel wall and helps differentiate between these two scenarios. These coronary evaginations are 10 times more common in first-generation than second-generation DESs.[23,24]

A radically different etiology for ST is the process of *neoatherosclerosis* evolving to plaque rupture or erosion and acute thrombus formation.[2,19,25] Unlike the previous scenarios, the stent struts are well covered with tissue in this case, and the thrombus originates from the exposed necrotic lipid core or from endothelial erosion. Neoatherosclerosis is a continuum of the spectrum of neointimal hyperplasia, where in addition to smooth muscle proliferation, lipid deposition, calcification, and intraplaque angiogenesis can occur, similar to a native coronary atherosclerotic plaque. By OCT, neoatherosclerosis typically has heterogeneous signal intensity with diffuse edges and high attenuation suggestive of lipid pools or sharply defined areas of signal attenuation suggestive of calcium deposition.[26] Plaque rupture is sometimes seen as a fissure in the neointimal fibrous cap with communication to the lipid pool.[27] Plaque rupture can occur spontaneously or as a consequence of stent fracture. ST due to neoatherosclerosis tends to occur late following stent implant,[28] unlike the prior scenarios of stent malapposition that are seen earlier.

It is important to point out that often a mix of the above pathologies can be identified inside the same thrombosed stent. The presence of thrombus is needed to indicate that the pathology is indeed the culprit for the clinical presentation. This is often possible even after multiple passes with aspiration catheters and limited angioplasty using small balloons (<2 mm).

6.4.3   Can OCT guide therapy in late or very late stent thrombosis?

An important observation emerging from the DESERT registry is the high risk of adverse clinical events following ST. In-hospital mortality was 3.8%, while the postdischarge major adverse cardiac event (MACE) rate was 16.4% and mortality was 2.8% at 12 months.[18] In the Dutch Stent Thrombosis Registry, which included acute and subacute ST, the mortality was even higher, with 1-year mortality at 10.7%.[17] Importantly, a large proportion of these events were due to recurrent problems in the same stent. Kubo et al. and Armstrong et al. reported a recurrent ST rate of 10.7% and TLR rate of 40%.[29,30]

The high risk of recurrence provides ample opportunity to improve the outcome of percutaneous treatment for ST. Given the diverse etiologies, OCT can offer a unique insight into the mechanism of the event and help guide therapy. In general, we advocate routinely performing OCT after aspiration thrombectomy, and occasionally after gentle balloon dilatation (<2 mm). In these acutely ill patients, restoration of flow is the primary objective and diagnostic imaging should be performed afterwards. Excessive thrombus burden may interfere with optimal imaging of the target segment due to dorsal shadowing. OCT can be performed with either manual or power injection of contrast, sometimes limiting the pullback length to the stented segment and the area of interest.

Interpretation of the OCT data in the acute setting should be done carefully, with a focus toward identifying the thrombus and its origin. Repeated aspiration thrombectomy is often necessary to improve image quality. The key questions the operator needs to address should include (1) whether the stent is well expanded and apposed, (2) whether the thrombus originates from an area of uncovered stent struts, and (3) whether significant neoatherosclerosis is present. As illustrated in the two case presentations, differentiation of late malapposition from neoatherosclerosis by OCT is usually straightforward.

What should be the default interventional treatment strategy for late or very late ST? Contemporary registries suggest that 60%–70% of these cases are treated with repeat stenting, while the remaining are treated with balloon dilatation alone.[31] The key concept underpinning the OCT-guided approach is that repeat indiscriminate stenting is unlikely to correct the causal problem and may in fact worsen the substrate for recurrent ST. In cases of stent malapposition, we advocate aggressive balloon dilatation to improve apposition, and the use of aggressive antithrombotic therapy with glycoprotein 2b/3a inhibitors to reduce the residual thrombus burden. Conceptually, it is unlikely that an additional layer of metal will decrease the likelihood of recurrent ST in this scenario. OCT can help us choose the appropriate balloon size to optimize stent apposition and expansion. On the other hand, a ruptured neoatherosclerotic plaque inside a stent is likely best treated with another stent, to seal dissections and improve lumen dimensions.

In conclusion, OCT can assist the interventionalist in identifying the underlying pathology associated with late or very late ST. Clinical data supporting the OCT-guided approach are currently lacking, but are certainly worthy of consideration. In patients with a high risk of recurrence, OCT can help guide the choice of further stenting in cases of neoatheroscleorosis versus aggressive balloon dilatation alone to correct strut malapposition.

REFERENCES

1. Buja LM. Vascular responses to percutaneous coronary intervention with bare-metal stents and drug-eluting stents: A perspective based on insights from pathological and clinical studies. *Journal of the American College of Cardiology* 2011;57(11):1323–6.
2. Nakazawa G et al. The pathology of neoatherosclerosis in human coronary implants bare-metal and drug-eluting stents. *Journal of the American College of Cardiology* 2011;57(11):1314–22.
3. Mehran R et al. Angiographic patterns of in-stent restenosis: Classification and implications for long-term outcome. *Circulation* 1999;100(18):1872–8.
4. Nakano M et al. Ex vivo assessment of vascular response to coronary stents by optical frequency domain imaging. *JACC Cardiovascular Imaging* 2012;5(1):71–82.
5. Kim JS et al. Long-term outcomes of neointimal hyperplasia without neoatherosclerosis after drug-eluting stent implantation. *JACC Cardiovascular Imaging* 2014;7(8):788–95.
6. Sakakura K, Joner M, Virmani R. Does neointimal characterization following DES implantation predict long-term outcomes? *JACC Cardiovascular Imaging* 2014;7(8):796–8.
7. Takano M et al. Appearance of lipid-laden intima and neovascularization after implantation of bare-metal stents extended late-phase observation by intracoronary optical coherence tomography. *Journal of the American College of Cardiology* 2009;55(1):26–32.
8. Kim JS et al. Quantitative and qualitative changes in DES-related neointimal tissue based on serial OCT. *JACC Cardiovascular Imaging* 2012;5(11):1147–55.
9. Kang SJ et al. Optical coherence tomographic analysis of in-stent neoatherosclerosis after drug-eluting stent implantation. *Circulation* 2011;123(25):2954–63.
10. Yonetsu T et al. Predictors for neoatherosclerosis: A retrospective observational study from the optical coherence tomography registry. *Circulation Cardiovascular Imaging* 2012;5(5):660–6.
11. Kang SJ et al. OCT-verified neoatherosclerosis in BMS restenosis at 10 years. *JACC Cardiovascular Imaging* 2012;5(12):1267–8.
12. Alfonso F et al. A randomized comparison of drug-eluting balloon versus everolimus-eluting stent in patients with bare-metal stent-in-stent restenosis: The RIBS V Clinical Trial (Restenosis Intra-stent of Bare Metal Stents: Paclitaxel-eluting Balloon vs. Everolimus-eluting Stent). *Journal of the American College of Cardiology* 2014;63(14):1378–86.
13. Byrne RA et al. Paclitaxel-eluting balloons, paclitaxel-eluting stents, and balloon angioplasty in patients with restenosis after implantation of a drug-eluting stent (ISAR-DESIRE 3): A randomised, open-label trial. *Lancet* 2013;381(9865):461–7.

14. Adriaenssens T et al. Optical coherence tomography study of healing characteristics of paclitaxel-eluting balloons vs. everolimus-eluting stents for in-stent restenosis: The SEDUCE (Safety and Efficacy of a Drug elUting balloon in Coronary artery rEstenosis) randomised clinical trial. *EuroIntervention* 2014;10(4):439–48.

15. Claessen BE et al. Stent thrombosis: A clinical perspective. *JACC Cardiovascular Interventions* 2014;7(10):1081–92.

16. Brodie BR et al. ST-segment elevation myocardial infarction resulting from stent thrombosis: An enlarging subgroup of high-risk patients. *Journal of the American College of Cardiology* 2012;60(19):1989–91.

17. van Werkum JW et al. Predictors of coronary stent thrombosis: The Dutch Stent Thrombosis Registry. *Journal of the American College of Cardiology* 2009;53(16):1399–409.

18. Waksman R et al. Correlates and outcomes of late and very late drug-eluting stent thrombosis: Results from DESERT (International Drug-Eluting Stent Event Registry of Thrombosis). *JACC Cardiovascular Interventions* 2014;7:1093–102.

19. Guagliumi G et al. Examination of the in vivo mechanisms of late drug-eluting stent thrombosis: Findings from optical coherence tomography and intravascular ultrasound imaging. *JACC Cardiovascular Interventions* 2012;5(1):12–20.

20. Finn AV, Otsuka F. Neoatherosclerosis: A culprit in very late stent thrombosis. *Circulation Cardiovascular Interventions* 2012;5(1):6–9.

21. Kotani J et al. Incomplete neointimal coverage of sirolimus-eluting stents: Angioscopic findings. *Journal of the American College of Cardiology* 2006;47(10):2108–11.

22. Inoue T et al. Impact of strut-vessel distance and underlying plaque type on the resolution of acute strut malapposition: Serial optimal coherence tomography analysis after everolimus-eluting stent implantation. *International Journal of Cardiovascular Imaging* 2014;30(5):857–65.

23. Räber L et al. Long-term vascular healing in response to sirolimus- and paclitaxel-eluting stents: An optical coherence tomography study. *JACC Cardiovascular Interventions* 2012;5(9):946–57.

24. Radu MD et al. Coronary evaginations are associated with positive vessel remodelling and are nearly absent following implantation of newer-generation drug-eluting stents: An optical coherence tomography and intravascular ultrasound study. *European Heart Journal* 2014;35(12):795–807.

25. Nakazawa G. Stent thrombosis of drug eluting stent: Pathological perspective. *Journal of Cardiology* 2011;58(2):84–91.

26. Takano M et al. Appearance of lipid-laden intima and neovascularization after implantation of bare-metal stents extended late-phase observation by intracoronary optical coherence tomography. *Journal of the American College of Cardiology* 2009;55(1):26–32.

27. Prati F et al. Expert review document on methodology, terminology, and clinical applications of optical coherence tomography: Physical principles, methodology of image acquisition, and clinical application for assessment of coronary arteries and atherosclerosis. *European Heart Journal* 2010;31(4):401–15.

28. Yonetsu T et al. Comparison of incidence and time course of neoatherosclerosis between bare metal stents and drug-eluting stents using optical coherence tomography. *American Journal of Cardiology* 2012;110(7):933–9.

29. Kubo S et al. Comparison of long-term outcome after percutaneous coronary intervention for stent thrombosis between early, late, and very late stent thrombosis. *Circulation Journal* 2014;78(1):101–9.

30. Armstrong EJ et al. Predictors and outcomes of recurrent stent thrombosis: Results from a multicenter registry. *JACC Cardiovascular Interventions* 2014;7(10):1105–13.

31. Yeo KK et al. Contemporary clinical characteristics, treatment, and outcomes of angiographically confirmed coronary stent thrombosis: Results from a multicenter California registry. *Catheterization and Cardiovascular Interventions* 2012;79(4):550–6.

Chapter 7

OCT assessment in spontaneous coronary artery dissection

Christopher Franco, Lim Eng, and Jacqueline Saw

7.1 SPONTANEOUS CORONARY ARTERY DISSECTION

7.1.1 Epidemiology

Spontaneous coronary artery dissection (SCAD) is a clinically challenging entity that is an important cause of both acute myocardial ischemia and infarction and sudden cardiac death, especially in women. The first case of SCAD was described on autopsy by Pretty et al. in 1931 of a 41-year-old woman presenting with sudden cardiac death who did not have risk factors for atherosclerotic disease.[1] The first angiographic report of SCAD was in 1973 by Forker et al. describing the angiographic appearance of extraluminal dye.[2] Since then, fewer than 1000 cases of SCAD have been noted in the medical literature. Retrospective registries have reported SCAD in 0.07%–1.1% of all coronary angiograms.[3–6] Previous reports have alluded to the rare observation of SCAD as a causative element in acute coronary syndrome (ACS) and sudden cardiac death, accounting for 0.1%–4% and 0.4%, respectively.[5,7] In a series by Vanzetto et al., the prevalence was higher among young women age <50, accounting for 8.7% of troponin-positive ACS.[3] We recently described a retrospective review of women under age 50 undergoing coronary angiography, and 24% had angiographically detectable SCAD.[1,8] Taken together, these data suggest that SCAD is much more prevalent than previously observed, but at present, the true population-based incidence of SCAD remains unknown.

There are several reasons to suspect that the incidence of SCAD has been underestimated in the medical literature. The association of SCAD with cardiac arrest may identify a small cohort of patients who die prior to presentation to hospital. Second, the inclusion of atherosclerotic coronary dissection, a mechanistically distinct variant from nonatherosclerotic SCAD (NA-SCAD), as it is currently defined, may have affected case definitions. Finally, given the often subtle clinical and angiographic presentation, many cases of SCAD have been misdiagnosed as mild atherosclerotic disease or missed altogether.

More recently, through meticulous angiographic review, we and others have described larger cohorts of patients with SCAD and identified SCAD as a far more prevalent cause of ACS in young women.[9–11] In a retrospective single-center cohort from the Mayo Clinic,[10] 87 angiographically confirmed cases of SCAD were identified, with 82% female and a mean age of 43 years. The initial clinical presentation was ST-elevation myocardial infarction (STEMI) in 49% of cases. SCAD recurred in 17%, with an estimated 10-year recurrence rate of 29%, underscoring the need for close follow-up. In the Madrid cohort,[9] a prospective series of 45 SCAD patients treated conservatively were followed for more than 6 years. Again, the majority were young (<50 years old) women presenting with acute MI. Interestingly, the predominant angiographic appearance of SCAD in this series was a long diffuse narrowing (type 2 angiographic SCAD—see below) rather than presenting as an intimal flap or vessel wall stain. Importantly, in those cases with angiographic follow-up, more than 50% of SCAD lesions had resolved with conservative therapy, underscoring the natural history of this disease and providing a clear rationale for conservative management.

We recently reported a large cohort of prospectively and retrospectively identified SCAD patients (n = 168).[11] In this report, 92% of patients were women (62% postmenopausal), with a mean age of 52. The dominant angiographic appearance of SCAD was again that of a smooth diffuse narrowing (type 2 angiographic SCAD) in 67% of cases. We examined the prevalence of potential predisposing conditions and demonstrated evidence of fibromuscular dysplasia (FMD) in 72%. Spontaneous angiographic SCAD "healing" was observed in 79/79 cases with angiographic follow-up, favoring a conservative management strategy in the majority of patients. Taken together, these more recent data identify SCAD as a clinically important cause of ACS in women, one that certainly should be considered in the differential diagnosis.

7.1.2   Pathogenesis

SCAD is defined as a nontraumatic and noniatrogenic separation of the coronary arterial wall by intramural hemorrhage and the resultant creation of a false lumen. The dissection plane can occur at the intimal–medial or medial–adventitial interface and need not have an intimal dissection flap.[12] The resulting intramural hematoma (IMH) can occlude or compromise the true vessel lumen, leading to myocardial ischemia and infarction.

There are two proposed mechanisms of SCAD. The first includes initiation of medial dissection and hemorrhage by an intimal tear and creation of a false lumen. The second involves the spontaneous development of an IMH, potentially due to disruption of the intra-arterial vasa vasorum.[13]

The etiology of SCAD is multifactorial, with contribution of both a predisposing arteriopathy (resulting in vulnerable vessel wall segments) and precipitating stressor events. Predisposing arteriopathies can be broadly classified as atherosclerotic SCAD (A-SCAD) and NA-SCAD.[11] Disruption of the atherosclerotic intima can lead to SCAD; however, these dissections tend to be limited in extent by medial atrophy and scarring.[14] Predisposing arteriopathies in NA-SCAD include peripartum arteriopathies (likely a culmination of hormonal exposure and hemodynamic changes during pregnancy), multiple previous pregnancies,[15] connective tissue disorders (e.g., Marfan's syndrome, Loeys–Dietz syndrome, Ehler–Danlos syndrome type 4, cystic medial necrosis, α-1 antitrypsin deficiency, and polycystic kidney disease), systemic inflammatory conditions (e.g., systemic lupus erythematosus, Crohn's disease, ulcerative colitis, polyarteritis nodosa, sarcoidosis, Churg–Strauss syndrome, Wegener granulomatosis, rheumatoid arthritis, Kawasaki, giant cell arteritis, and celiac disease), coronary spasm, or idiopathic arteriopathies.[11]

The predominance of female sex in the SCAD population may speak to a mechanistic role for hormonal status in its pathogenesis, and earlier reports of SCAD proposed an association with pregnancy and oral contraceptive use.[16,17] While recent series have challenged this notion, estrogen level and pregnancy status remain important risk factors for SCAD, but their exact contribution to the pathogenesis of SCAD remains unclear.[11,18]

Precipitating stress events increase shear forces locally and may precipitate SCAD in vulnerable vessel segments. Precipitating events identified in SCAD have included intense exercise (isometric or aerobic), intense emotional stress, labor and delivery, intense valsalva-type activities (e.g., retching, vomiting, bowel movement, and coughing), sympathomimetic drugs (e.g., cocaine, amphetamines, and methamphetamines), and intense hormonal therapy (e.g., β-human chorionic gonadotropin [HCG] injections). In our series, more than half of patients who presented with SCAD reported a precipitating stressor.[11]

The relative frequency of predisposing and precipitating factors in the pathogenesis remains an area of active investigation. We recently reported a large SCAD cohort and identified several predisposing arteriopathies, with the most prevalent being FMD (72%), idiopathic arteriopathies (20.1%), and hormonal therapy (10.7%).[11]

7.1.3 Fibromuscular dysplasia

FMD is a segmental nonatherosclerotic, noninflammatory vasculopathy of the small to medium-sized arteries that can affect all layers of the vessel wall. Historically, FMD was classified histologically into intimal fibroplasia, medial fibroplasia (correlating with the angiographic string of beads appearance), perimedial fibroplasia, and adventitial fibroplasia.[19,20] Case reports have demonstrated severe disorganization of the ultrastructure of the arterial wall with alternating areas of smooth muscle cell hyperplasia and adventitial collagen deposition with loss of the anatomical boundaries of the elastic lamellae, all contributing to severe luminal obstruction. The first case of coronary FMD associated with SCAD was reported in 1987 by autopsy.[19] Multiple case reports, including our own, have since implicated coronary FMD as a central predisposing arteriopathy in the pathogenesis of SCAD.[11,19,21–27] Interestingly, intracoronary imaging with intravascular ultrasound (IVUS) and optical coherence tomography (OCT) has the ability to document areas of bright, echogenic and reflective collagen interspersed with areas of cellular hyperplasia (Figure 7.1), similar to the histological descriptions of FMD.[24]

Angiographically, coronary FMD may appear with the classical description of medial fibroplasia with a string of beads appearance, but this is relatively infrequent.[28] More likely, coronary FMD may angiographically appear normal, as small arterioles may be involved, with suspected microvascular dysfunction. Other coronary angiographic appearances are diffuse stenosis, tubular stenosis, and ectasia. In addition, in patients presenting with overlying SCAD on preexisting FMD, the standard acute angiographic appearance of SCAD may be observed (see description below). This appearance normalizes with resorption of the IMH that occurs with healing of the dissection.

The diagnosis of coronary FMD remains challenging, and much of the data supporting an association between FMD and SCAD have emerged from the incidental detection of renal and iliofemoral FMD

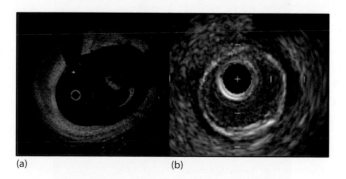

(a)   (b)

Figure 7.1 Intracoronary images of patients with suspected coronary FMD. (a) OCT image of a patient showing a thickened fibrotic intimal–medial layer from six to two o'clock, with the more prominent darker deeper layer likely representing hyperplasia; and (b) IVUS image of a different patient showing circumferential bright dual fibrotic intimal layers or internal elastic lamina, surrounded by thick echolucent media.

observed during routine coronary angiography. Our group described the first series of SCAD with incidental FMD.[26,29] Furthermore, in our initial cohort of 50 SCAD patients, 86% of them had concomitant renal, ilio-femoral, or cerebrovascular FMD.[8] These findings were supported by previous reports[10] noting an association with iliofemoral FMD in cases of SCAD. In our updated large 168-patient SCAD series, we detected FMD in 72% of cases.[11] Given the prevalence of this association, we suspect that previous cases of idiopathic SCAD may have had underlying undiagnosed FMD.

7.1.4 Angiographic features of SCAD: saw angiographic SCAD classification

The two-dimensional luminogram offered by traditional angiography is indispensable for the rapid evaluation of patients with acute myocardial ischemia. However, the main limitation of angiography is its inability to visualize the layers of the coronary vessel wall. The diagnosis of SCAD relies on often subtle angiographic features, and careful attention to vessel opacification and stenosis characterization is critical to help differentiate IMHs from other causes of coronary stenosis. The administration of intra-arterial vasodilators is important to rule out the contribution of arterial spasm to subtle narrowings. As patients with SCAD often have generalized coronary arterial fragility, a cautious and meticulous approach to performing coronary angiography is advised, for example, avoiding catheter dampening, deep catheter engagements, and forceful injections.

Early identification of SCAD is paramount in the management of patients presenting with ACS, as the therapeutic strategy differs significantly from that for atherosclerotic stenosis. Coronary angiography provides two-dimensional assessment of coronary anatomy and flow. It remains the mainstay of investigation in patients with suspected SCAD. Pathognomonic angiographic appearances may include multiple radiolucent lines, a false lumen, contrast staining, and late contrast clearing, all of which are consistent with an intimal tear. Saw proposed three distinctive angiographic patterns to improve the diagnostic accuracy of SCAD.[30] Type 1 (evident arterial wall stain) has the characteristic angiographic appearance, as described, and is easily detected on coronary angiography (Figure 7.2). Type 2 (diffuse stenosis of varying severity) involves predominantly mid- to distal segments with a subtle but abrupt change in vessel caliber. It typically appears

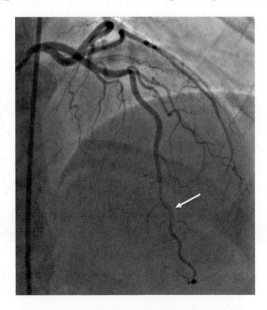

Figure 7.2 Type 1 angiographic SCAD (according to angiographic classification by Saw criteria) of the distal left anterior descendent artery (LAD) with contrast arterial wall stain (arrow).

diffuse (usually >20 mm) and with smooth narrowing (Figure 7.3). This is the most common form of SCAD, accounting for about two-thirds of cases.[11] Type 3 (mimic atherosclerosis) is essentially indistinct from atherosclerotic stenosis on coronary angiography and is virtually impossible to diagnose without the adjunctive use of intracoronary imaging (Figure 7.4). It may have suggestive features, such as long lesions (11–20 mm), hazy or linear stenosis, and the absence of atherosclerotic changes in other coronary arteries.[30]

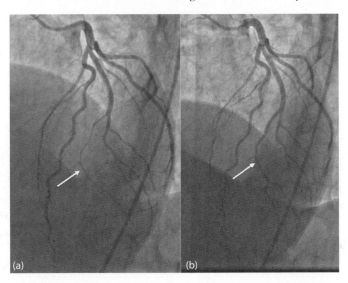

Figure 7.3 Type 2 angiographic SCAD (Saw criteria). (a) Mid- to distal segment of a large diagonal branch (arrow) and (b) spontaneous angiographic healing of this diagonal branch on repeat angiogram 1 year later (arrow).

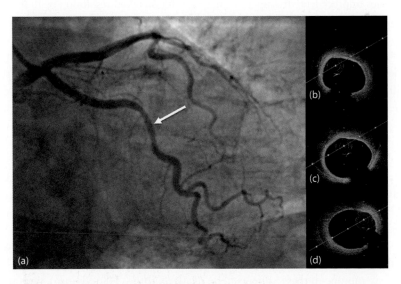

Figure 7.4 Type 3 angiographic SCAD (Saw criteria) with (a) the angiogram showing moderate 60% stenosis of the mid–circumflex artery (arrow), but OCT showing an IMH; (b) a crescent-shaped false lumen filled with an IMH from seven to four o'clock; (c) a crescent-shaped false lumen with an IMH of heterogeneous reflexivity due to the heterogeneity of coagulated blood in the false lumen, with full extent of the IMH well visualized from seven to twelve o'clock; and (d) an edge of the dissected artery with a thin crescent-shaped IMH from eight to one o'clock.

7.1.5 Intracoronary imaging of SCAD

By virtue of its inability to visualize the coronary arterial wall, traditional angiography limited diagnostic accuracy in SCAD.[5,6] Intracoronary imaging with tomographic techniques, including IVUS[13] and OCT,[31] can provide a direct assessment of the ultrastructure of the arterial wall and its intimal–medial contents. IVUS has a spatial resolution of 150 μm with deeper tissue penetration, and while it cannot identify intimal tears well, it can readily identify IMHs as a homogenous collection behind an intimal–medial membrane.[32] By contrast, OCT generates three-dimensional images from optical scattering within tissue and has a spatial resolution of 10–15 microns.[33,34] On OCT images, fibrous tissue and collagen appear bright (high reflectivity), while areas of smooth muscle hyperplasia or hematoma appear dark (low reflectivity).[24,35] OCT has significant advantages over IVUS in the diagnosis of SCAD due to the superior spatial resolution, and can differentiate clearly between IMHs and lipid-rich or calcified atheromata,[31,35,36] and identify intimal tears or entry sites of dissection. Given the superiority of OCT imaging for SCAD diagnosis, this modality will be reviewed in detail in the next section.

7.2 ROLE OF OCT IN THE DIAGNOSIS AND MANAGEMENT OF SPONTANEOUS CORONARY ARTERY DISSECTION

The development of OCT has revolutionized the diagnosis of patients with SCAD, which has been challenging, especially for those without type 1 angiographic appearance. OCT is a novel intracoronary imaging modality utilizing the principle of reflected light for the generation of intraluminal images. Since its first introduction in 1991,[37] it has gained popularity as a diagnostic tool in various medical specialities, including coronary intervention. Near-infrared light of 1250–1350 nm wavelength is aimed at a target, and subsequently the resulting intensity and echo time delay from the reflected light are measured by interferometer for image acquisition. It produces unprecedentedly superior image resolution (axial resolution of 10 μm and lateral resolution of 20 μm), allowing comprehensive visualization and assessment of the coronary anatomy and pathology.

The limitations of coronary angiography in diagnosing SCAD were alluded to previously. Alfonso and colleagues reported that only 3 patients out of 11 patients with confirmed SCAD on OCT had an intimal flap on coronary angiography.[31] This is also collaborated by a more contemporary case series recently published showing that <30% of patients with SCAD had classical type 1 angiographic appearances.[11] This largely explains the underdiagnosis of SCAD in the past, compounded by the lack of appropriate intracoronary imaging and knowledge of this clinical entity at the time. Moreover, type 2 and 3 SCADs are easily missed using conventional angiography.

OCT has proven to be an invaluable imaging modality in guiding the diagnosis of patients with suspected SCAD.[31,35,38,39] It facilitates the visualization of an IMH, double lumen, and dissection flap at the intimal–medial interface, which are readily defined on OCT (Figure 7.5). In the prospective series of SCAD diagnosed with OCT by Alfonso et al.,[31] 17 cases with features suspicious for SCAD on traditional angiography were assessed by OCT, and 11 (82% female, mean age 48) had confirmed SCAD. The characteristic double lumen was seen in all cases; however, only 3/11 had a distinct intimal flap or entry point, with the remainder showing only an IMH without an intimal flap. All patients had associated thrombus in either true or false lumens. They also found the intimal–medial membrane in these patients to be relatively thick (348 ± 84 μm), with the thinnest part of the intimal–medial membrane at the edges of the intimal tear.[31] OCT also allows for the detailed assessment and identification of the precise origin of intimal disruption, the length of the affected vessel, the thickness and distribution of the dissection flap, the magnitude of luminal compromise, side branch involvement, and associated thrombus formation. All this information is valuable when planning coronary intervention.

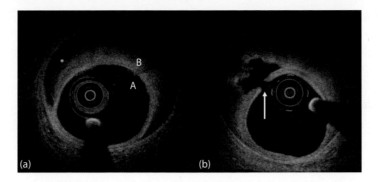

Figure 7.5 OCT images showing (a) an IMH (*) and double lumen (A, true lumen; B, false lumen) and (b) intimal tear (arrow).

Nevertheless, since the majority of SCAD cases may be managed conservatively without percutaneous coronary intervention (PCI), the dominant role of OCT in this condition is simply to make the diagnosis of SCAD. For this purpose, the OCT catheter need not be placed across the full length of the dissection. In our practice, the OCT catheter imaging tip is placed at the beginning of the suspected dissected segment, and a "live-view" image is then assessed to look for an IMH. If the catheter is not occlusive, we then perform contrast injection to activate the pullback.

In our proposed diagnostic algorithm (Figure 7.6), early coronary angiography should be offered to all patients with suspected SCAD. Type 1 SCAD is readily identified by angiography alone. In the absence of this pathognomonic angiographic appearance, OCT or IVUS is recommended for further assessment. In patients who display type 2 appearance, intracoronary nitroglycerine should be administered to eliminate

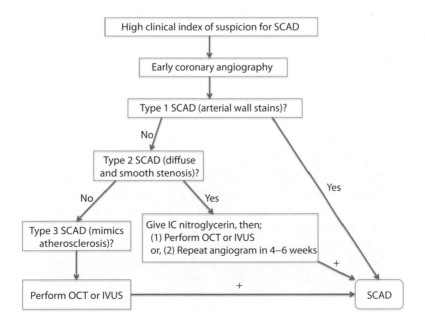

Figure 7.6 Suggested diagnostic algorithm for SCAD diagnosis. IC, intracoronary. (From Saw, J., *Circ. Cardiovasc. Interv.*, 84, 1115–1122, 2014. Reproduced with permission.)

the possibility of coronary spasm. If this appearance persists, intracoronary imaging should be performed if the diagnosis is uncertain, or alternatively, coronary angiography can be repeated 4–6 weeks later to confirm the diagnosis when angiographic healing occurs. Type 3 appearances should always be investigated with intracoronary imaging, as they are practically indistinct to atherosclerosis angiographically.[30]

7.2.1 OCT guidance for PCI

PCI in patients with SCAD is technically demanding and challenging. Wiring the true lumen poses the risk of propagation of the dissection plane, while deploying a coronary stent at the false lumen is potentially disastrous. In these circumstances, OCT is essential in providing unique anatomical and morphological insights, which would otherwise be missed using conventional angiography. Under direct visualization, OCT confirms the positioning of the angioplasty wire in the true lumen, accurate localization of the intimal disruption site, and the full extent of the IMH involved to facilitate stent sizing and length and deployment. Adequate apposition of deployed stent struts is readily assessed using OCT (Figure 7.7a), and this is important to avoid late stent thrombosis related to malapposition. This risk can be increased with acquired malapposition following resorption of the IMH with dissection healing (Figure 7.7b).

The main limitation encountered when using OCT is the necessity to establish a blood-free environment during imaging. Dissected intimal flaps are generally fragile and at risk of further extension. There are concerns that contrast flushes, even at a minimal amount and force, may generate considerable hydraulic pressure to propagate axial dissection and compromise coronary flow distally. However, this risk appears theoretical, and we have not encountered complications related to hydraulic dissection in our small series of SCAD with intracoronary imaging.[40] Another limitation with OCT is the poor depth of tissue penetration (1–2.5 mm), which can result in failure to depict the entire thickness of the dissected plane and IMH. Significant shadowing caused by red thrombus in the false lumen may in turn degrade the quality of the generated images. However, these limitations should not significantly limit the utility of OCT during PCI, which should predominantly entail true lumen access, dissection length assessment, and stent strut apposition.

IVUS is an alternative form of intracoronary imaging frequently used in clinical practice. It uses a concept that relies on the emission and backscattering of ultrasonic waves to convert to electrical signals in order to generate images. However, the resolution of IVUS is by far inferior to that of OCT (axial resolution of 150 μm). The effectiveness of IVUS in diagnosing SCAD without characteristic angiographic features was first described by Maehara et al. in 2002 when he successfully identified five patients who had medial dissection related to an IMH in the absence of a concomitant intimal tear.[41] Similarly, Arnold et al. also validated

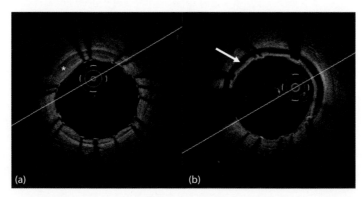

Figure 7.7 OCT images showing (a) stent strut apposition during acute stent procedure (*) and (b) gaps behind the stent struts at the intermediate 2-week follow-up due to resorption of the IMH (arrow).

its clinical implication in the diagnosis of four patients with SCAD.[32] Overall, IVUS is useful to confirm the presence of an IMH and double lumen, and identify the true lumen and severity of luminal compression; however, it may miss visualizing intimal tears when compared with OCT (Figure 7.5).

Although there are complementary roles of OCT and IVUS in SCAD imaging, the cost of both imaging modalities precludes simultaneous use in most laboratories. Despite its superior imaging resolution, OCT is insufficient in tissue penetration, preventing detailed assessment of the full thickness of the dissection plane involved. Most of the outer border of the vessel wall will be poorly visualized. On the other hand, IVUS, with its higher tissue penetration strength (10 mm), allows evaluation of the external elastic lamina and the entire extent of dissected segments, even in patients with large-caliber coronary vessels or intraluminal red thrombus.[38] In a prospective study conducted by Paulo and colleagues, they examined the combined use of OCT and IVUS in the assessment of patients with SCAD. They demonstrated the superiority of OCT in the recognition of intimal ruptures and intraluminal thrombi. A false lumen and IMH were well elucidated; however, the full depth and extent of IMH could not be determined due to shadowing interference and inadequate penetration. This was easily overcome by concomitant use of IVUS, which provided complete vessel visualization with the assessment of a significantly longer diseased segment and larger false lumen areas. Thrombus with heterogeneous appearance in the false lumen is readily illustrated on IVUS.[42,43] Poon and colleagues also illustrated the successful utilization of this combination in guiding PCI.[43]

7.3 MANAGEMENT OF SCAD

The optimal management and medical therapy for SCAD is unknown and is largely empirical in the absence of any randomized studies. Apart from anecdotal reports on clinical outcomes, there is also little evidence-based guidance on criteria for revascularization or methods therein. A high index of clinical suspicion in an appropriate context is crucial and may preempt the use of unnecessary and potential harmful therapies. As serial angiographic reports have supported the notion that the natural history of SCAD includes complete healing in patients managed without intervention, a conservative management strategy is appropriate in most cases.[9–11] We previously reported a simple management algorithm regarding the need for revascularization according to the clinical status of patients presenting with SCAD (Figure 7.8).[11] Revascularization for SCAD should be considered in patients with active myocardial ischemia or hemodynamic instability. PCI should be considered in patients with localized proximal dissections in large vessels associated with ongoing ischemia or reduced thrombolysis in myocardial infarction (TIMI) flow. Coronary artery bypass grafting (CABG) should be reserved for patients with left main or multivessel proximal large-vessel dissection, especially in the setting of hemodynamic compromise. However, graft patency failure after resolution of the IMH and restoration of native coronary flow has been reported, presumably due to competitive flow in the native arteries.[10,11]

With regard to medical management, we have previously published a review of available literature.[1] We advocate routine long-term therapy with aspirin and a beta-blocker following SCAD presentation, if tolerated. We are conducting a small prospective randomized trial to evaluate the use of statins and angiotensin-converting enzyme (ACE) inhibitors in the SAFER-SCAD study, which will hopefully provide some guidance on the management of this condition.

PCI in SCAD is associated with significant technical difficulties attributed to the fragility of the vessel wall. Technical difficulties might include guidewire placement in the true lumen, dissection in small-caliber distal vessels, risk of dissection propagation, and side branch occlusion. Care must be taken to avoid stent

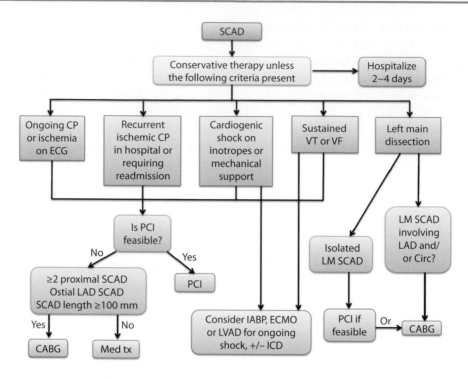

Figure 7.8 Recommended management algorithm. CP, chest pain; ECG, electrocardiogram; VT, ventricular tachycardia; VF, ventricular fibrillation; Tx, treatment; IABP, intraaortic balloon pump; ECMO, extracorporeal membranous oxygenation; LVAD, left ventricular assist device; Circ, circulation. (From Saw, J. et al., *Circ. Cardiovasc. Interv.*, 7, 645–655, 2014. Reproduced with permission.)

or vessel overdilation, which may lead to propagation of the dissection or perforation.[27] In addition, SCAD segments frequently require long stent length, increasing the risk of restenosis. Direct stenting may be preferable over predilation when possible, and the stent placement can be guided by OCT. Some groups[9,44] have protocolized OCT-guided stent deployment at the proximal and distal ends of the dissection prior to stenting the middle to mitigate IMH propagation. Finally, the temporal resolution of an IMH in previously stented segments may increase the risk of late stent malapposition and in-stent thrombosis.[18] In all cases, avoiding overstenting and "full metal jacket" is important. The use of bioabsorbable stents in SCAD is theoretically appealing, since it both allows local "sealing" of the dissection entry site and addresses the problem of late stent malapposition after resorption of the residual IMH.

Multiple reports have identified generally poor technical results post-PCI. In our recent cohort of 168 patients, 33 underwent PCI, with 12/33 (36%) being unsuccessful. Of successful or partially successful PCI, 57% had extension of dissection, with 6%, 24%, and 12% demonstrating stent thrombosis, restenosis, or a CABG requirement, respectively. Overall, the number of PCIs with a durable successful result was a meager 30%.[11] These findings are supported by previous reports demonstrating 35% failure of PCI in SCAD.[8,10] Interestingly, a radial approach may be associated with an increased risk of iatrogenic dissections in SCAD patients, with 3/41 radial angiograms resulting in iatrogenic dissection secondary to deep intubation of the left main coronary ostium. By contrast, no dissections were noted in the patients with femoral access.[11] Clearly, meticulous angiographic techniques are crucial in the complex population, with particular attention to avoiding deep intubation and pressure damping, and gentle contrast injection.

7.4 FUTURE DIRECTIONS

The addition of OCT to the interventional cardiologists' armamentarium has fundamentally changed our ability to diagnose and manage SCAD. Through the identification of new cases, unparalleled visualization of its pathogenesis, and ability to evaluate the local effect of novel therapies, OCT continues to provide novel insight into important disease. Of note, the recent reporting of micro-OCT, a three-dimensional imaging technique with unprecedented 1- to 2-micron spatial resolution, has the potential to provide subcellular insight into the *in vivo* vascular biology of vulnerable vessel segments possibly prior to their dissection.[45] For instance, in patients with coexisting FMD, it will be remarkable to evaluate the coronary artery for histological FMD changes adjacent to dissected segments, to better understand the mechanism predisposing to SCAD. Despite these advances, a major hurdle in this field remains the paucity of randomized data and evidence-based guidelines to direct the care of this complex patient population. Further prospective studies of long-term outcome and defining the optimal medical therapy are sorely needed.

7.5 CONCLUSIONS

In summary, SCAD is an infrequent condition that has been underdiagnosed and misdiagnosed. Usage of intracoronary imaging with IVUS or OCT improves the accurate diagnosis of this challenging condition. Diagnostic and management algorithms have been recently proposed to improve the diagnosis and therapeutic stratification of this condition. OCT has superior spatial resolution that is unparalleled in modern-day commercially available imaging technology. This imaging modality is instrumental in the diagnosis of SCAD cases where angiographic findings are ambiguous for confirming SCAD. Understanding the role and appropriate utilization and careful use of this technology is expected to improve the diagnosis of SCAD, as well as the outcomes with PCI if clinically indicated.

REFERENCES

1. Saw J. Spontaneous coronary artery dissection. *Canadian Journal of Cardiology* 2013;29:1027–33.
2. Forker AD et al. Primary dissecting aneurysm of the right coronary artery with survival. *CHEST Journal* 1973;64:656–8.
3. Vanzetto G et al. Prevalence, therapeutic management and medium-term prognosis of spontaneous coronary artery dissection: Results from a database of 11,605 patients. *European Journal of Cardio-Thoracic Surgery* 2009;35:250–4.
4. Shamloo BK et al. Spontaneous coronary artery dissection: Aggressive vs. conservative therapy. *Journal of Invasive Cardiology* 2010;22:222.
5. Mortensen KH et al. Spontaneous coronary artery dissection: A Western Denmark Heart Registry study. *Catheterization and Cardiovascular Interventions* 2009;74:710–7.
6. Vrints C. Spontaneous coronary artery dissection. *Heart* 2010;96:801–8.
7. Hill SF, Sheppard MN. Non-atherosclerotic coronary artery disease associated with sudden cardiac death. 2010;96:1119–25.
8. Saw J et al. Spontaneous coronary artery dissection: Prevalence of predisposing conditions including fibromuscular dysplasia in a tertiary center cohort. *JACC Cardiovascular Interventions* 2013;6:44–52.
9. Alfonso F et al. Spontaneous coronary artery dissection: Long-term follow-up of a large series of patients prospectively managed with a "conservative" therapeutic strategy. *JACC Cardiovascular Interventions* 2012;5:1062–70.
10. Tweet MS et al. Clinical features, management, and prognosis of spontaneous coronary artery dissection. *Circulation* 2012;126:579–88.
11. Saw J et al. Spontaneous coronary artery dissection: Association with predisposing arteriopathies and precipitating stressors and cardiovascular outcomes. *Circulation Cardiovascular Interventions* 2014;7:645–55.

12. Reynolds H. Mechanisms of myocardial infarction without obstructive coronary artery disease. *Trends in Cardiovascular Medicine* 2014;24:170–6.

13. Maehara A et al. An intravascular ultrasound classification of angiographic coronary artery aneurysms. *American Journal of Cardiology* 2001;88:365–70.

14. Isner JM et al. Attenuation of the media of coronary arteries in advanced atherosclerosis. *American Journal of Cardiology* 1986;58:937–9.

15. Vijayaraghavan R et al. Clinician update: Pregnancy-related spontaneous coronary artery dissection. *Circulation* 2014;130:1915–20.

16. Koul AK, Hollander G, Moskovits N. Coronary artery dissection during pregnancy and the postpartum period: Two case reports and review of literature. *Catheterization and Cardiovascular Interventions* 2001;52:88–94.

17. Giacoppo D et al. Spontaneous coronary artery dissection. *International Journal of Cardiology* 2014;175:8–20.

18. Alfonso F et al. Spontaneous coronary artery dissection. *Circulation Journal* 2014;78:2099–110.

19. Lie JT, Berg KK. Isolated fibromuscular dysplasia of the coronary arteries with spontaneous dissection and myocardial infarction. *Human Pathology* 1987;18:654–6.

20. Harrison EG Jr, McCormack LJ. Pathologic classification of renal arterial disease in renovascular hypertension. *Mayo Clinic Proceedings* 1971;46(3):161–7.

21. Brodsky SV et al. Ruptured cerebral aneurysm and acute coronary artery dissection in the setting of multivascular fibromuscular dysplasia: A case report. *Angiology* 2008;58:764.

22. Mather PJ, Hansen CL, Goldman B. Postpartum multivessel coronary dissection. *Journal of Heart and Lung Transplantation* 1993;13(3):533–7.

23. Saw J et al. Nonatherosclerotic coronary artery disease in young women. *Canadian Journal of Cardiology* 2014;30:814–9.

24. Saw J, Poulter R, Fung A. Intracoronary imaging of coronary fibromuscular dysplasia with OCT and IVUS. *Catheterization and Cardiovascular Interventions* 2013;82:E879–83.

25. Garcia NA et al. Spontaneous coronary artery dissection: A case series and literature review. *Journal of Community Hospital Internal Medicine Perspectives* 2014;4.

26. Pate GE, Lowe R, Buller CE. Fibromuscular dysplasia of the coronary and renal arteries? *Catheterization and Cardiovascular Interventions* 2005;64:138–45.

27. Poulter R, Ricci D, Saw J. Perforation during stenting of a coronary artery with morphologic changes of fibromuscular dysplasia: An unrecognized risk with percutaneous intervention. *Canadian Journal of Cardiology* 2013;29:519.e1–3.

28. Michelis K et al. Coronary artery manifestations of fibromuscular dysplasia. *Journal of the American College of Cardiology* 2014;64:1033–46.

29. Saw J et al. Spontaneous coronary artery dissection in patients with fibromuscular dysplasia: A case series. *Circulation Cardiovascular Interventions* 2012;5:134–7.

30. Saw J. Coronary angiogram classification of spontaneous coronary artery dissection. *Catheterization and Cardiovascular Interventions* 2014;84:1115–22.

31. Alfonso F et al. Diagnosis of spontaneous coronary artery dissection by optical coherence tomography. *Journal of the American College of Cardiology* 2012;59:1073–9.

32. Arnold JR et al. The role of intravascular ultrasound in the management of spontaneous coronary artery dissection. *Cardiovascular Ultrasound* 2008;6:24.

33. Abtahian F, Jang I-K. Optical coherence tomography: Basics, current application and future potential. *Current Opinion in Pharmacology* 2012;12:583–91.

34. Alfonso F, Canales E, Aleong G. Spontaneous coronary artery dissection: Diagnosis by optical coherence tomography. *European Heart Journal* 2009;385.

35. Lim C, Banning A, Channon K. Optical coherence tomography in the diagnosis and treatment of spontaneous coronary artery dissection. *Journal of Invasive Cardiology* 2010;22:559–60.

36. Prati F et al. Expert review document on methodology, terminology, and clinical applications of optical coherence tomography. *European Heart Journal* 2010;31:401–15.

37. Huang D et al. Optical coherence tomography. *Science* 1991;254:1178–81.

38. Alfonso F, Paulo M, Dutary J. Endovascular imaging of angiographically invisible spontaneous coronary artery dissection. *JACC Cardiovascular Interventions* 2012;5:452–3.

39. Ishibashi K, Kitabata H, Akasaka T. Intracoronary optical coherence tomography assessment of spontaneous coronary artery dissection. *Heart (British Cardiac Society)* 2009;95:818.

40. Saw J et al. Angiographic appearance of spontaneous coronary artery dissection with intramural hematoma proven on intracoronary imaging. *Journal of the American College of Cardiology* 2014;64:B3.

41. Maehara A et al. Intravascular ultrasound assessment of spontaneous coronary artery dissection. *American Journal of Cardiology* 2002;89:466–8.

42. Paulo M et al. Combined use of OCT and IVUS in spontaneous coronary artery dissection. *JACC Cardiovascular Imaging* 2013;6:830–2.

43. Poon K et al. Spontaneous coronary artery dissection: Utility of intravascular ultrasound and optical coherence tomography during percutaneous coronary intervention. *Circulation Cardiovascular Interventions* 2011;4:e5–7.

44. Walsh SJ, Jokhi PP, Saw J. Successful percutaneous management of coronary dissection and extensive intramural haematoma associated with ST elevation MI. *Acute Cardiac Care* 2008;10:231–3.

45. Liu L et al. Imaging the subcellular structure of human coronary atherosclerosis using micro-optical coherence tomography. *Nature Medicine* 2011;17:1010–14.

Chapter 8

Optical coherence tomography assessment for cardiac allograft vasculopathy after heart transplantation

Sameer J. Khandhar and Guilherme Oliveira

8.1 INTRODUCTION

8.1.1 Background

Heart transplantation remains the definitive therapy for patients with advanced congestive heart failure. Approximately 5000 transplants are performed every year worldwide, with the number remaining stable over the past decade due to limitations of donor availability.[1] Early posttransplant survival has improved, but median survival remains 10.4 years, with cardiac allograft vasculopathy (CAV) as the leading cause of graft failure and second leading cause of death in patients beyond 3 years after transplantation.[1]

CAV is now often considered the "Achilles' heel" of transplantation due to the poor prognosis it portends and its often silent progression until an advanced disease state. CAV is an unfortunately common problem after transplantation, with 18% of patients developing it by year 1 and more than 50% by 10 years.[2] CAV accounts for 10%–14% of deaths beyond 1 year after transplantation, with the cause of death attributable to heart failure from graft dysfunction, arrhythmias, or sudden death.

Autopsy studies in transplant recipients with established CAV demonstrate that CAV is a combination of intimal fibromuscular hyperplasia, traditional atherosclerosis, and vasculitis, with intimal hyperplasia of the small and large coronary arteries being the most common finding.[3] A small degree of intimal thickening due to a longitudinal layer of smooth muscle cells exists beneath the endothelium in normal nontransplanted coronary arteries; however, in CAV, the neointima also consists of a new layer of connective tissue, mononuclear cells, and smooth muscle cells covered by the traditional thin endothelial cell layer. This progressive thickening of the neointimal layer is the hallmark feature of CAV and is what causes gradual lumen narrowing.[4] In this chapter, we review the importance of screening and the pathophysiology of CAV, and further explore the utilization of optical coherence tomography (OCT) as a novel and ideal imaging tool for this disease process.

8.2 SCREENING AND DIAGNOSING CAV

We review in detail the variety of ways to screen and diagnose CAV first, prior to discussing the pathophysiology, so that sample images can be shown with a better understanding.

Screening and diagnosing CAV presents a difficult clinical dilemma since most patients with CAV are asymptomatic due to cardiac sensory denervation resulting from the transplant surgery. This prevents the development of typical angina symptoms despite progressive coronary lumen narrowing and ischemia. Therefore, being able to screen patients for subclinical disease is of the utmost importance.

A noninvasive stress test is designed to detect flow-limiting coronary obstruction and is not effective for early detection when intimal hyperplasia has yet to cause significant luminal narrowing. Angiography is the most common method of screening, and what the current grading system is based on, however, is of limited value since it visualizes only luminal diameter and cannot image the coronary vessel wall to detect intimal hyperplasia. The sensitivity of coronary angiography alone for CAV is suboptimal and may lead to underestimation of the true disease burden given the diffuse nature of the disease and lack of a normal reference.[5–7] Despite the inability to detect early CAV lesions, angiography and stress testing provide important prognostic information by assessing for obstructive CAV.[5] Other modalities, such as computed tomography angiography (CTA), magnetic resonance imaging (MRI), and even blood testing, are under investigation but have not yet become part of routine clinical care.

Due to these limitations, intravascular imaging with intravascular ultrasound (IVUS) and virtual histology IVUS were appealing and well studied over the past 10–20 years. While these offer additional information compared with angiography, they are still limited by their resolution of 100–300 microns. Therefore, these methods cannot accurately measure or characterize the neointima layer alone, and can only assess the entire wall thickness (intima and media). Using IVUS, progression of intima + media thickness to greater than 500 μm is associated with poor outcomes[8–10]; however, the resolution of IVUS does not allow for measuring subtle changes that may impact outcomes, and manual measurements do not correlate well with automated software.[11] By the time CAV is detectable by angiography or IVUS, it tends to be more advanced, and therefore not surprisingly associated with worse outcomes.[8] IVUS is not able to quantify mild–moderate amounts of CAV as accurately, and therefore may not fully predict the natural progression and outcomes in milder or early CAV.

OCT allows for high-resolution imaging of the coronary architecture and accurate measurements for intimal thickness and plaque characterization, which is appealing. Several small studies have now shown the utility of OCT in this disease process, and we will explore this further throughout the chapter.

8.3 CAV PATHOPHYSIOLOGY

Although not completely understood, it is thought that the pathogenesis of CAV involves repeated injuries to the endothelium from a variety of factors, such as cellular-mediated rejection, alloimmune factors, ischemia–reperfusion injury at the time of transplant, cytomegalovirus (CMV) infection, immunosuppression medications, systemic inflammation, and traditional atherosclerosis risk factors,[5,7,12,13] as listed in Table 8.1. A schematic and theoretical progression of disease is illustrated in Figure 8.1. Damage to the endothelium leads to smooth muscle cell proliferation, infiltration of the intima with inflammatory cells, and collagen deposition.[14] This process causes the evolution from focal intimal thickening early after transplant to circumferential diffuse thickening and development of atherosclerotic plaques at later stages.[15,16] The absolute amount of intimal hyperplasia tends to be constant in the entire arterial tree but is more noticeable in the distal

TABLE 8.1

CAV risk factors

Donor-derived factors

    Older age or male donor

    Donor CAD

    Donor HTN/LVH

    Explosive donor death

Recipient-derived factors (nonmodifiable)

    Older recipient age

    Male recipient

    History of ischemic heart disease

    VAD support prior to OHT

    Infection prior to OHT

Recipient metabolic factors (modifiable)

    HTN

    Hyperlipidemia

    Insulin resistance/diabetes

    Smoking

    Higher body mass index

Immunologic factors

    Cyclosporine use (instead of tacrolimus)

    Azathioprine instead of mycophenolate

    Cellular-mediated rejection

    Antibody-mediated rejection

    CMV infection

Note: HTN, hypertension; LVH, left ventricular hypertrophy; VAD, ventricular assist device; OHT, orthotopic heart transplant.

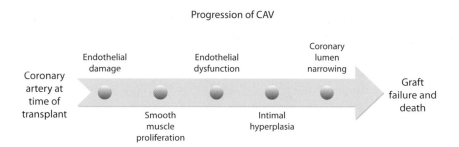

Figure 8.1   Theoretical progression of CAV.

vasculature given the smaller lumen size.[17,18] The composition of the intimal layer can change over time and with disease progression, as illustrated in Figure 8.2. Early intimal hyperplasia likely represents mononuclear cell infiltration and smooth muscle cell proliferation, whereas in advanced CAV, the intimal layer becomes progressively more solid and results in a fibrous layer that likely is irreversible.[4] This progression is illustrated in Figure 8.3.

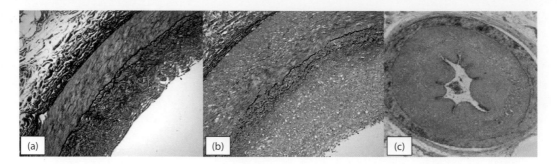

Figure 8.2 Pathology slides representing various degrees of CAV. (a) Histological appearance of coronary artery immediately after transplant with equal intimal and medial thickness. (b) Progression of intimal hyperplasia. (c) Severe intimal hyperplasia resulting in lumen loss. (Reprinted from Huibers, M.M.H. et al. *Atherosclerosis*, 236, 353–359, 2014; Arbustini, E., and Roberts, W.C., Am. J. Cardiol., 78, 814–820, 1996.)

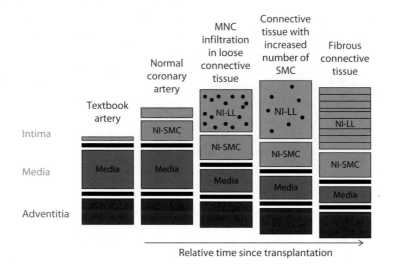

Figure 8.3 Schematic representation of the various phenotypes of CAV NI-LL, neointima luminar layer; NI-SMC, neointima smooth muscle cell layer; MNC, mononuclear cell. (Reprinted from Huibers, M.M.H. et al., *Atherosclerosis*, 236, 353–359, 2014.)

8.3.1 Role of rejection

Rejection of the transplanted heart is an immunologic response against the donor and a risk factor for developing CAV. Cellular rejection mediated by T cells plays a larger role than the humoral system as far as we currently know.

Donor antigens present on the transplanted heart, including the endothelium of the coronary arteries, activate recipient T cells through antigen-presenting cells. Once there is immune activation, T cells, macrophages, and plasma cells infiltrate the heart, leading to myocyte injury and death. Rates of cellular rejection are lower now with advances in peritransplant induction and immunosuppressive therapies but remain an important risk factor for developing CAV.

The development of CAV, however, is much more complex than simply being due to significant or even low levels of chronic cellular rejection. The role of the humoral immune system and how antibody-mediated injury leads to CAV is just starting to be understood and is felt to be significant.[19,20] The host immune response against donor human leukocyte antigen (HLA), non-HLA, and endothelial antigens can lead to damage to the coronary endothelium of the transplanted heart. Roughly 9% of patients who undergo transplantation are sensitized to HLA antibodies (panel reactive antigen >10%) at the time of the transplant. Clinical outcomes in these patients are worse because of increased rejection and CAV.[1] It is recognized that even patients with a negative cross-match at the time of transplant can develop *de novo* donor-specific antibodies (DSAs) to HLAs and non-HLAs after transplantation, which may play a role in the development of CAV. There is no way to predict who will develop these antibodies if they are not present at the time of transplant, and studies remain ongoing on how to best treat patients with DSAs.

8.3.2   Traditional atherosclerosis

Beyond intimal hyperplasia, atherosclerotic coronary lesions, including lipophilic and calcified plaques, can also occur. These atherosclerotic plaques may already be present in the donor heart at the time of transplantation or develop *de novo* afterwards. Preexisting plaques at the time of transplant can rapidly progress afterwards, leading to focal stenosis that usually affects the proximal portions of the major epicardial coronary arteries.[14] The influence of traditional atherosclerotic risk factors, such as older donor age, hypertension, left ventricular hypertrophy, and donor coronary disease, emphasizes the overlapping pathophysiology.[6,13,21,22] Early CAV, defined as within the first year of heart transplantation, reflects either progression of donor-derived coronary artery disease (CAD) (especially focal, proximal lesions) or an aggressive CAV phenotype that behaves like an inflammatory vasculitis. Although preexisting donor-derived atherosclerosis can become clinically significant, whether all such plaques will progress is not fully understood.

8.4   OCT UTILIZATION POST–HEART TRANSPLANTATION

OCT is theoretically an ideal coronary imaging tool for the detection of early neointimal hyperplasia since high-resolution imaging is needed for accurate characterization of the intima and media layers, and since deep tissue penetration is not required.[23] Due to this superior resolution, OCT can detect very early neointimal hyperplasia, and it accurately tracks its progression over time. Since OCT is still a relatively novel tool, the long-term prognostic data that we have with stress testing, angiography, and IVUS do not yet exist for OCT. As OCT use becomes more widespread and more studies are performed, these data should become available.

There have been several separate series published on the use of OCT after heart transplantation. While none of these unfortunately have been directly compared with histology, the high-resolution findings are consistent with prior autopsy-based studies.

OCT imaging has been performed by standard technique with the commercially available C7-XR system from St. Jude Medical by automated pullback with simultaneous injection of contrast for clearance of blood. The mid–left anterior descending artery (LAD) has been most commonly studied, and performing OCT imaging in transplant patients does not appear to carry any additional risk.

8.4.1   Intimal hyperplasia

The existing studies illustrate that the intimal and medial layers of the coronary arteries in transplant patients could be measured reliably by OCT, and that between 50% and 70%[17,24] of patients had CAV by OCT, often despite normal coronary angiography. Figure 8.4 illustrates the OCT findings of normal coronary artery versus one with significant CAV, including how to measure the intima and medial layers separately. The superior resolution of OCT allows for distinct identification of the internal and external elastic membranes

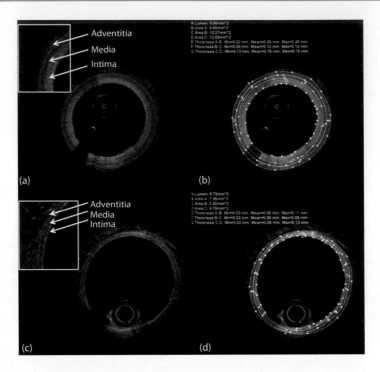

Figure 8.4 OCT images and sample measurements of the layers of the coronary artery in a patient with CAV (a and b) and a patient without CAV (c and d).

by high-backscattering bands. Being able to trace the lumen and intimal and medial layers allows for detailed analysis of variables such as lumen area, intimal thickness, media thickness, intimal volumes, and total plaque volumes (defined as intima + media volume, similar to IVUS studies).

In this group of patients, the difficulty resides in defining a threshold for abnormal intimal thickening. The normal coronary endothelium and intima are thin layers residing on the internal elastic membrane. Despite the notion that the intima is a single cell layer, autopsy studies have shown the normal intima to have some degree of hyperplasia, and that in patients with CAV there is a second layer of immune-mediated hyperplasia on top.[4] These studies also confirmed that the intimal hyperplasia tends to be a diffuse process, affecting from the distal to proximal vessels uniformly, and that the intimal layer thickens while the media layer undergoes only small changes despite disease progression.

8.4.2 Atherosclerotic plaques

Traditional atherosclerosis likely plays a role in graft failure and death, in addition to intimal hyperplasia. Patients with advanced CAV causing graft failure requiring retransplantation were frequently noted to have traditional atherosclerosis on gross pathology.[3]

In addition to intimal hyperplasia, detection of lipid-rich and calcified atherosclerotic plaques was reported in up to 50%–60% of patients. Plaques tended to be noted in focal areas of intimal hyperplasia, and sample images of lipid-rich and calcified plaques are illustrated in Figure 8.5. Lipid-rich regions are defined as an area of low signal with poorly defined margins and signal attenuation or shadowing behind the plaque. Calcified regions were identified as sharply delineated areas of decreased signal with significant signal attenuation, as described in earlier chapters.

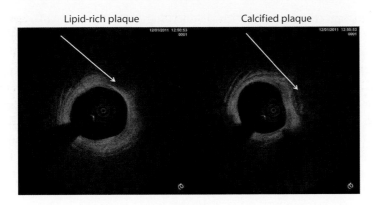

Figure 8.5 OCT images to represent lipid-rich and calcified coronary plaques identified after transplantation.

Complicated coronary lesions, including vulnerable plaques with thin-cap, intimal laceration, intraluminal thrombus, macrophage infiltration, and side branch involvement, and layered complex plaque, were also noted on detailed analysis. These atherosclerotic findings were more prevalent several years after transplantation, suggesting the development of new plaque and not donor derived. Sample OCT images of these findings are demonstrated in Figure 8.6.

Thin-cap atheroma is defined as a lipid-rich plaque covered by a thin fibrous cap that is <65 microns in thickness. Macrophages are defined as signal-rich distinct punctate regions on the plaque surface and are typically

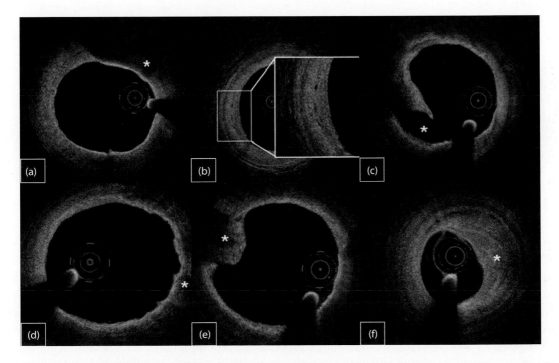

Figure 8.6 OCT representations of complex plaque after transplantation. (a) Lipid-rich plaque with thin cap. (b) Microchannels. (c) Plaque rupture. (d) Intimal laceration without rupture. (e) Thrombus. (f) Layers of plaque leading to lumen obstruction.

associated with attenuation (Figure 8.6a). Microchannels suggestive of neovascularization within the intimal hyperplasia are defined as distinct signal-poor voids that can be followed for several consecutive frames (Figure 8.6b). Plaque rupture is characterized as a disruption of the intimal cap (Figure 8.6c), and along the same spectrum is intimal laceration, that is, unevenness of the intimal layer without obvious rupture (Figure 8.6d). Thrombus is defined as a mass-like structure attached to the intima on the lumen side (Figure 8.6e), and finally, layered plaque has the appearance of heterogeneous regions within the intima in a layered pattern (Figure 8.6f).[24]

This constellation of findings of intimal laceration, presence of macrophages, and layered plaque suggests that plaque erosion, rather than plaque rupture, is the mechanism for thrombus formation and progression. Despite these findings in a large percentage of patients, their clinical implications are not fully understood since acute coronary syndromes and total occlusion of coronary arteries are very rare in CAV, with most cases involving progressive diffuse narrowing of the coronary arteries. Therefore, larger prospective studies are necessary to truly determine the significance of these plaques.

8.4.3 Correlation with cellular rejection

In a study by Dong et al., 48 patients underwent OCT imaging after transplant and OCT findings were compared by rejection history. In the 11 patients who had high-grade rejection, the mean intimal thickness was significantly greater (350 microns versus 140 microns). In addition to the intimal hyperplasia seen in patients with a history of rejection, the group with a history of rejection had a higher incidence of intimal microvessels, intimal calcification, intraluminal thrombus, and even plaque rupture.[18]

8.4.4 Comparison with IVUS

IVUS has been utilized after transplantation to study CAV since the 1990s, and therefore there are several large prospective studies to provide insight into disease progression and prognosis. These IVUS-based studies have clearly shown a worse prognosis once there is intimal thickness of greater than 500 microns, which is not surprising since this represents a severe form of CAV. However, the impact of early intimal hyperplasia not detectable by the resolution of IVUS is not known, and further OCT studies are required to answer this.

Hou et al., in a letter to the editor, described OCT use compared with IVUS in a small cohort of patients and found that OCT detected intimal thickness, defined as >100 microns, in 66% of patients, while IVUS only detected intimal hyperplasia in 14%.[25] Cassar et al. found a strong correlation ($r = 0.85$) between IVUS and OCT for the detection of CAV in 53 patients with more significant intimal hyperplasia who had an average intima + media thickness of 600 microns. At this degree of severe disease, there is no surprise that both IVUS and OCT can detect CAV.[24]

The greatest benefit of OCT appears to reside in the ability to detect the early and subtle changes of CAV, in addition to detecting atherosclerotic plaques, as seen in Figure 8.7, which illustrates a case of early intimal hyperplasia with a thickness of about 150 microns that was not detected by angiography or IVUS.

Characterization of plaque has been attempted with IVUS and virtual histology IVUS in the past,[26–28] but when done by De la Torre Hernandez for this purpose, only 14% of patients could have reliable assessment for atherosclerosis because the intimal hyperplasia that usually accompanies plaque further decreased the resolution. OCT, on the other hand, not only allows for characterization in all patients despite intimal hyperplasia but also can characterize the plaque in great detail. Imamura et al.[29] report a case of layered complex plaque in which OCT imaging identified two layers of intimal hyperplasia likely representing donor atherosclerosis with superimposed intimal hyperplasia that occurred after transplantation. IVUS correctly identified thickening of the combined intimal and medial layers but does not have the resolution to further characterize the intimal layer in detail.

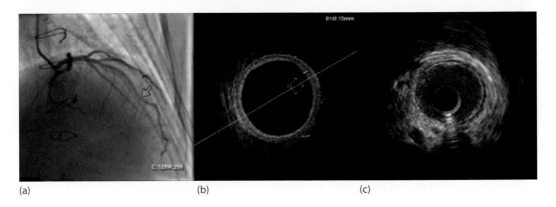

(a)   (b)   (c)

Figure 8.7 Detection of intimal thickening by OCT in a patient with normal angiogram and IVUS images. (a) Quantitative coronary angiography revealed a 14% diameter stenosis. (b) OCT revealed intimal hyperplasia with a thickness of 150 microns. (c) Accurate measurement of intimal hyperplasia was difficult with IVUS.

8.5 TREATMENT OF CAV

The field of heart transplantation has grown tremendously since the first heart transplant in 1967 by Christian Barnard. Despite these advances, CAV remains one of the leading causes of graft failure. Newer immunosuppression agents[30] and traditional atherosclerotic risk factor modification, especially with the utilization of statins, seem to have a beneficial impact.[31] Revascularization with stenting or bypass surgery remains an option for patients with focal disease, and retransplantation remains the only definitive treatment for advanced CAV with graft dysfunction.

The data obtained by OCT, imaging including early intimal hyperplasia and plaque characterization, may offer insight and allow for earlier treatment. Theoretically, the early treatment of intimal hyperplasia before there is extensive fibrosis of the intimal layer and treatment of unstable plaque or thrombus with traditional atherosclerotic agents, such as statins and aspirin, may allow for higher success rates. While the role of OCT in guiding therapy and altering the natural history remains speculative, ongoing studies will hopefully help answer these questions.

8.6 CONCLUSION

OCT allows for accurate high-resolution quantitative imaging of the coronary arteries and characterization of intimal hyperplasia and atherosclerotic plaques. OCT imaging has allowed for *in vivo* assessment of findings previously noted only on autopsy studies and has extended our understanding of CAV beyond just intimal hyperplasia to also involving complex atherosclerotic plaques. The clinical significance of these findings, and whether early detection and treatment ultimately improve outcomes, is not known and remains to be seen with future studies.

REFERENCES

1. Stehlik J et al. The registry of the International Society for Heart and Lung Transplantation: Twenty-seventh official adult heart transplant report—2010. *Journal of Heart and Lung Transplantation* 2010;29:1089–103.

2. Prada-Delgado O et al. Prevalence and prognostic value of cardiac allograft vasculopathy 1 year after heart transplantation according to the ISHLT recommended nomenclature. *Journal of Heart and Lung Transplantation* 2012;31:332–3.
3. Lu WH et al. Diverse morphologic manifestations of cardiac allograft vasculopathy: A pathologic study of 64 allograft hearts. *Journal of Heart and Lung Transplantation* 2011;30:1044–50.
4. Huibers MMH et al. Distinct phenotypes of cardiac allograft vasculopathy after heart transplantation: A histopathological study. *Atherosclerosis* 2014;236:353–9.
5. Colvin-Adams M, Agnihotri A. Cardiac allograft vasculopathy: Current knowledge and future direction. *Clinical Transplantation* 2011;25(2):175–84.
6. Zimmer RJ, Lee MS. Transplant coronary artery disease. *JACC Cardiovascular Interventions* 2010;3:367–77.
7. Schmauss D, Weis M. Cardiac allograft vasculopathy: Recent developments. *Circulation* 2008;117:2131–41.
8. Kobashigawa JA et al. Multicenter intravascular ultrasound validation study among heart transplant recipients. *Journal of the American College of Cardiology* 2005;45:1532–7.
9. Li H et al. Vascular remodeling after cardiac transplantation: A 3-year serial intravascular ultrasound study. *European Heart Journal* 2006;27:1671–7.
10. Tuzcu EM et al. Intravascular ultrasound evidence of angiographically silent progression in coronary atherosclerosis predicts long-term morbidity and mortality after cardiac transplantation. *Journal of the American College of Cardiology* 2005;45:1538–42.
11. D'Errico V et al. Reproducibility of IVUS measurements in heart transplant recipients: Increased quality of data by using dedicated software for image analysis. *Computers in Cardiology* 2008;35:537–40.
12. Arora S et al. Systemic markers of inflammation are associated with cardiac allograft vasculopathy and an increased intimal inflammatory component. *American Journal of Transplantation* 2010;10:1428–36.
13. Rahmani M et al. Allograft vasculopathy versus atherosclerosis. *Circulation Research* 2006;99:801–15.
14. Van Loosdregt J et al. The chemokine and chemokine receptor profile of infiltrating cells in the wall of arteries with cardiac allograft vasculopathy is indicative of a memory T-helper 1 response. *Circulation* 2006;114:1599–607.
15. Starnes VA et al. Cardiac transplantation in children and adolescents. *Circulation* 1987;76:V43–7.
16. Tuzcu EM et al. Dichotomous pattern of coronary atherosclerosis 1 to 9 years after transplantation: Insights from systematic intravascular ultrasound imaging. *Journal of the American College of Cardiology* 1996;27:839–46.
17. Khandhar SJ et al. Optical coherence tomography for characterization of cardiac allograft vasculopathy after heart transplantation (OCTCAV study). *Journal of Heart and Lung Transplantation* 2013;32:596–602.
18. Dong L et al. Optical coherence tomographic evaluation of transplant coronary artery vasculopathy with correlation to cellular rejection. *Circulation Cardiovascular Interventions* 2014;7:199–206.
19. Michaels PJ et al. Humoral rejection in cardiac transplantation: Risk factors, hemodynamic consequences and relationship to transplant coronary artery disease. *Journal of Heart and Lung Transplantation* 2003;22:58–69.
20. Caforio AL et al. Immune and nonimmune predictors of cardiac allograft vasculopathy onset and severity: Multivariate risk factor analysis and role of immunosuppression. *American Journal of Transplantation* 2004;4:962–70.
21. Stehlik J et al. The Registry of the International Society for Heart and Lung Transplantation: 29th official adult heart transplant report—2012. *Journal of Heart and Lung Transplantation* 2012;31:1052–64.
22. Stehlik J et al. The Registry of the International Society for Heart and Lung Transplantation: Twenty-eighth adult heart transplant report—2011. *Journal of Heart and Lung Transplantation* 2011;30:1078–94.
23. Prati F et al. Expert review document on methodology, terminology, and clinical applications of optical coherence tomography: Physical principles, methodology of image acquisition, and clinical application for assessment of coronary arteries and atherosclerosis. *European Heart Journal* 2010;31:401–15.
24. Cassar A et al. Coronary atherosclerosis with vulnerable plaque and complicated lesions in transplant recipients: New insight into cardiac allograft vasculopathy by optical coherence tomography. *European Heart Journal* 2013;34:2610–7.
25. Hou J et al. OCT assessment of allograft vasculopathy in heat transplant recipients. *JACC Cardiovascular Imaging* 2012;5:662–3.
26. De la Torre Hernandez JM et al. Virtual histology intravascular ultrasound assessment of cardiac allograft vasculopathy from 1 to 20 years after transplantation. *Journal of Heart and Lung Transplantation* 2009;28:156–62.
27. Torres HJ et al. Prevalence of cardiac allograft vasculopathy assessed with coronary angiography versus coronary vascular ultrasound and virtual histology. *Transplantation Proceedings* 2011;43:2318–21.
28. Konig A et al. Assessment of early atherosclerosis in de novo heart transplant recipients: Analysis with intravascular ultrasound-derived radiofrequency analysis. *Journal of Heart and Lung Transplantation* 2008;27:26–30.

29. Imamura T et al. Cardiac allograft vasculopathy can be distinguished from donor-transmitted coronary atherosclerosis by optical coherence tomography imaging in a heart transplantation recipient: Double layered intimal thickness. *International Heart Journal* 2014; 55: 178–80.

30. Eisen H et al. Everolimus versus mycophenolate mofetil in heart transplantation: A randomized multicenter trial. *American Journal of Transplantation* 2013;13:1203–16.

31. Kobashigawa JA et al. Ten-year follow-up of a randomized trial of pravastatin in heart transplant patients. *Journal of Heart and Lung Transplantation* 2005;24:1736–40.

Chapter 9

OCT assessment out of the coronary arteries

Jun Li, Daniel Kendrick, Vikram S. Kashyap, and Sahil A. Parikh

9.1 INTRODUCTION

Peripheral arterial disease (PAD) affects 20% of the population over the age of 65.[1–3] The presence of PAD not only serves as an important surrogate for the development of coronary artery disease, but also can have a profound effect on the quality of life in patients with claudication. Dr. Thomas Fogarty and Dr. Charles Dotter independently introduced endovascular therapies in the peripheral vasculature in the 1960s with the use of balloon catheter angioplasty.[4–8] Endovascular techniques are now widely used by vascular surgeons, interventional cardiologists, and interventional radiologists in the peripheral vasculature. Although conventional angiography provides information in the two-dimensional plane of the vessel outline and luminal dimension, it lacks detail regarding lesion morphology and vessel wall characteristics. Intravascular imaging serves as a useful adjunct to traditional angiography in the characterization and treatment of vascular disease.

9.2 HISTORY OF INTRAVASCULAR IMAGING

The evolution of intravascular imaging began with the introduction of intravascular ultrasound (IVUS) in 1972.[9] Its initial *in vivo* application in the United States was in the coronary system in the late 1980s, while its use in peripheral vascular beds was popularized in the 1990s.[5,10–12] IVUS in the peripheral vasculature has several applications, including assessment of a culprit lesion's composition and dimensions to guide treatment decisions, along with evaluation of the quality of a treated lesion.[10]

Two mechanisms are available for IVUS image acquisition: solid-state dynamic aperture and mechanical scanning. In the solid-state method, transducer elements are positioned circumferentially around the catheter tip and are activated sequentially to acquire an array of images.[10,11] The mechanical system is composed of an ultrasound transducer at the tip of a flexible, high-torque catheter on which it rotates.

The resolution of IVUS is dependent on the frequency of the ultrasound catheter, with higher frequencies providing improved resolution, but at the cost of decreased penetration distance. In the peripheral vascular bed, frequencies between 8 and 12 mHz are used for larger vessels, such as the aorta, inferior vena cava, and iliac aneurysms.[10] A higher frequency of 20 mHz is appropriate for imaging of smaller vessels, such as an occlusive iliac artery, or the femoral, infrapopliteal, carotid, and renal arteries.[10] Frequencies of 20–45 mHz allow for spatial resolution of 200–500 μm, whereas 10 mHz provides a spatial resolution of 150 μm.[10,13]

The gray-scale echo signals can help differentiate between layers of the arterial wall and plaque composition. Both the intima and adventitia appear bright and echogenic, while the media is echolucent. It may be difficult to discern the adventitia from the surrounding tissue.[13] Lesion constituents (calcific, fibrotic, and lipid-rich plaques) and distribution (eccentric and concentric) can be important in the determination of the response to treatment and may help dictate treatment modality. On ultrasound, calcium will appear bright with posterior shadowing, while lipid appears echolucent. Fibrous plaques are also echogenic but lack the posterior shadowing of calcific lesions.

The advent of color flow and three-dimensional (3D) reconstruction has been useful in the differentiation between luminal flows from echolucent mural structures, and to identify dissection planes. Unlike echocardiography and color Duplex sonography, where color flow is obtained from the Doppler effect, the color flow in IVUS is generated by computer software based on differences (i.e., movement of blood particles) detected between two sequential adjacent frames.[14] The images acquired are displayed as axial planes and 3D longitudinal reconstructions. Due to different acquisition techniques, color flow by IVUS cannot provide information on flow velocities.

To assist with planning for interventions, direct intraluminal measurements allow for appropriate determination of the minimal luminal area in the normal vasculature that flanks the lesion of interest, with the goal of determining the appropriate sizing of an interventional device, such as a balloon or stent. However, longitudinal reconstruction with IVUS is not accurate, partly due to tortuous vessels causing distortion when constrained into a straight path and partly due to long acquisition times. This may overall limit the ability to precisely predict the stent length necessary for treatment.[10] Due to the acquisition techniques of IVUS, limitations exist in its ability to assess lesion dimensions and plaque constituents, and thus alternative imaging modalities have been developed.[15]

9.3 OPTICAL COHERENCE TOMOGRAPHY

Optical coherence tomography (OCT) was initially introduced in the 1990s, with its first utilization in optical imaging.[16] It is currently widely used in ophthalmology, dermatology, gastroenterology, and interventional cardiology.[16] It has been fully integrated into the clinical imaging of the coronary vascular beds, with demonstrated utility in the characterization of atherosclerotic lesions, as well as assistance with stent deployment. The full scope of these intracoronary uses is covered elsewhere in this text.

9.3.1 Comparison with IVUS

Similar to IVUS, OCT is based on the concept of reflected energy to generate cross-sectional intravascular images, with changes in time delay and intensity dependent on tissue composition. Unlike IVUS, which uses acoustic signals as the source of energy, OCT emits low coherence light, or near-infrared light, as its source.

Due to the significantly faster speed of light (3.0×10^8 m/s, compared with the speed of sound at 1.5×10^3 m/s), OCT requires the use of a reference arm and an interferometer to acquire the backscatter of light and echo delays in order to generate an image of the vessel wall.[17] The first-generation time-domain OCT (TD-OCT) imaging system entailed use of a single frequency emission and a moving reference mirror, rendering image procurement to occur at a rate of 1 mm/s.[15,17] Due to its relatively long image acquisition time, proximal balloon occlusion was required during pullback in order to adequately clear blood from the region of interest. Furthermore, there were limited radial fields of view, which resulted in underestimation of luminal diameter compared with IVUS and precluded application to vessels >3.75 mm in diameter.[15,17]

The current generation of frequency- or Fourier-domain OCT (FD-OCT) emits multiple frequencies simultaneously (aka frequency swept) with a reference mirror that is fixed. Faster pullbacks at ≥20 mm/s, as well as increased luminal scan diameter, permit imaging of vessels up to 10 mm in size.[18] These factors have allowed for OCT imaging in larger-caliber peripheral vessels with longer, multifocal lesions using a nonocclusive flush technique. Rather than occlude proximal flow, a flush medium is used to briefly clear blood from the imaged region during catheter pullback. A detailed explanation of how each of these OCT systems function and their associated advantages are addressed elsewhere in this text.

In contrast to IVUS, OCT offers a spatial resolution that is greater than 10 times more powerful, with an axial resolution of 10–20 μm and a lateral resolution of 25–30 μm, providing significantly higher-fidelity image quality.[10,15,17,19] Furthermore, the frame rate is higher (100 fps, compared with 30 fps in IVUS) and the pullback rate is faster (≥20 mm/s in FD-OCT, compared with 0.5–1 mm/s in IVUS), both of which allow for significantly faster image acquisition.[10,16]

Limitations of OCT are tissue penetration depth, maximal vessel size that can be imaged, and unique imaging artifacts. Due to scattering and absorption of light beams within biological tissues, OCT is limited to tissue penetration depths of 0.5–2.0 mm, compared with 10 mm in IVUS. Imaging artifacts particular to OCT include suboptimal flushing with residual blood obscuring the field of view, nonuniform rotational distortion, sew-up or seam-line artifact, fold-over artifact, and saturation artifact; these are addressed in detail elsewhere in this text.[10,17]

9.3.2 Technique

To date, three published series of peripheral OCT imaging studies in the superficial femoral artery (SFA) have used FD-OCT systems.[20–22] Flush medium was used for blood clearance in these studies, although one group also included proximal femoral manual occlusion to assist in image acquisition. Our typical technique for image capture in the SFA is described here.

At our institution, we utilize the ILUMIEN OPTIS and OPTIS Integrated Systems (St. Jude Medical, Minneapolis, Minnesota) with the Dragonfly OPTIS Imaging Catheter (St. Jude Medical). This catheter consists of a single fiber-optic wire mounted within a fluid-filled cylinder with a 0.019 in. external diameter. A lens assembly at the distal aspect reflects emitted light at an angle nearly perpendicular to the fiber itself. Percutaneous access is obtained in the common femoral artery contralateral to the lesion of interest. A 6F introducer sheath is first inserted, and access is obtained to the ipsilateral common iliac artery with the use of a 5F universal flush (UF) catheter. Depending on vessel characteristics on initial diagnostic images, a combination of standard 0.018–0.035 in. guidewires and hydrophilic catheters are used to gain access to the region of interest. We usually advance a crossover sheath approximately 10 cm from the lesion of interest, to ensure focused directional delivery of the flush media during image pullback. The crossing wire is then exchanged for a 0.014 in. wire, on which the monorail system for OCT can be loaded.

The media used for image optimization should be optically transparent and efficient in blood clearance. Iodinated contrast is presently the preferred modality of flush media in the coronary arena. This allows for the concomitant acquisition of an angiogram during an OCT recording. In the PAD literature, a variety of media have been utilized.[18,21]

In a recently published cohort study from our center, OPTical Imaging Measurement of Intravascular Solution Efficacy (OPTIMISE), four types of flush media were analyzed for quality of blood clearance and image acquisition: heparinized saline, iodinated contrast, dextran, and carbon dioxide (CO_2).[20] Each of these

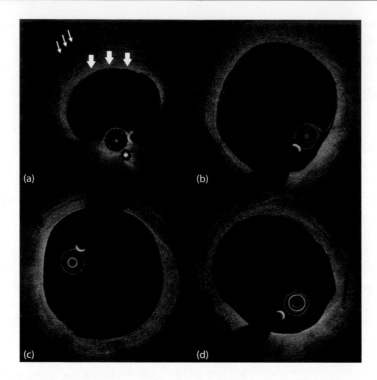

Figure 9.1 Representative OCT findings using various forms of flush media in one patient, within the same region of interest in the SFA. (a) CO_2 has previously been used as a noncontrast alternative for angiographic assessment in the peripheral vasculature. Under OCT, CO_2 retains its gaseous form (gas bubble, asterisk) and provides limited washout of the intraluminal space, creating pseudostenoses (broad arrows). The true arterial wall (narrow arrows) is obscured by residual intraluminal blood. OCT under (b) iodinated contrast, (c) dextran, and (d) heparinized saline provides similar washout and quality of images.

is an optically transparent medium, with iodinated contrast and dextran having indexes of refraction closest to human plasma and theoretically ideal at mitigating any artifact from residual blood during the flush. In the lower extremity, CO_2 has been used for many years in conjunction with digital subtraction angiography in patients at risk for contrast-related kidney injury.[23,24] Head-to-head qualitative comparisons of each of these media demonstrated that heparinized saline, dextran, and iodinated contrast were all comparable in SFA OCT imaging, whereas CO_2 was significantly inferior to images acquired with heparinized saline. This is suspected to be due to the retention of CO_2 as gas bubbles during the injection, resulting in the production of pseudostenoses. Figure 9.1 illustrates the representative findings on OCT using different types of flush media.

At our institution, the preferred flush media is diluted iodinated contrast to minimize irritation to the lower extremity during injection of undiluted contrast alone, and yet angiographic image acquisition can still be obtained simultaneously for lesion characterization.

9.4 CLINICAL APPLICATIONS OF OCT IN THE PERIPHERAL VASCULATURE

Despite the widespread acceptance of OCT in the coronary vasculature, there has been scant work to date in exploring the role of OCT in the peripheral circulation. The currently preferred modality of intravascular assessment in the PAD arena remains IVUS.[10] Nonetheless, OCT offers a number of advantages over IVUS due to image acquisition techniques, and should be considered as an alternative adjunct by endovascular peripheral interventionalists.

The following examples serve as an atlas of lesion pathologies identified by using OCT in the peripheral vasculature. The accompanying case vignettes illustrate the important clinical applications of this high-resolution intravascular imaging modality in the lower extremities. Multiple pathologies can coexist in one patient, and the vignettes will be revisited as the atlas progresses from diagnostic to interventional findings.

9.4.1 Diagnostic utilization: lesion characterization

9.4.1.1 Fibrotic and lipid-rich plaques: case 1

A 54-year-old woman with diabetes, hypertension, dyslipidemia, and panvascular atherosclerosis manifesting as coronary disease requiring prior left anterior descending stent placement and a history of stroke presents with complaints of lifestyle-limiting claudication of the left lower extremity.

Her peripheral angiography shows focal left SFA stenosis with a single-vessel runoff via the posterior tibial artery, with reconstitution of the anterior tibial at the foot. A cross section of the stenotic segment is consistent with fibrotic plaque with underlying calcific lesions (Figure 9.2a). Proximal to the stenosis, the presence of lipid-rich plaques is appreciated (Figure 9.2b). A lumen profile is created with OCT, which helps with determination of the reference vessel diameter and lesion length to plan for an interventional strategy (Figure 9.3a).

9.4.1.2 Calcified plaques: case 2

A 70-year-old man with coronary artery disease, diabetes, and tobacco use presents with progressively debilitating bilateral lower extremity claudication. His peripheral angiogram shows subtotal occlusion of the proximal right SFA and otherwise diffuse, heavily calcified disease throughout the SFA (Figure 9.2c). The popliteal artery is widely patent with two-vessel runoff via the anterior and posterior tibial arteries.

Light penetrates calcium, which accounts for the low-signal (dark) plaques with low signal attenuation (deep penetration of light beyond calcium). These tend to have discrete borders. Conversely, lipid-rich plaques have diffuse and irregular borders with high signal attenuation, causing limited visualization of the underlying tissue. Fibrotic plaques tend to be high signal (bright) with low attenuation.[17]

9.4.1.3 In-stent restenosis: case 3

A 58-year-old man with hypertension, stroke, nonischemic cardiomyopathy, and PAD with prior right-sided lower extremity rest pain requiring placement of a right SFA self-expanding nitinol stent. The patient returns to the office 7 months later with recurrent right-sided claudication symptoms. Duplex ultrasound is suggestive of in-stent restenosis (ISR). Angiography with concomitant OCT pullback demonstrates severe, diffuse neointimal hyperplasia (NIH) (Figure 9.2d). The lumen profile recapitulates the severity and extent of restenosis (Figure 9.3b).

The use of conventional angiography allows for generalized quantification of ISR as diffuse, focal, or edge related.[25] With the advent of OCT, significant details, such as the presence of neoatherosclerosis and neovascularization, can be identified.[25,26] In the coronary vasculature, neointimal characteristics may portend differences in major adverse cardiac event-free survival.[27] The clinical implications of these findings in the peripheral vasculature are yet to be elucidated.[22]

9.4.1.4 Vein graft: case 4

A 65-year-old woman with previous femoral–tibial venous bypass presents with recurrent claudication and is found to have a high-grade stenosis after the distal anastomosis on ultrasound. Angiography demonstrates

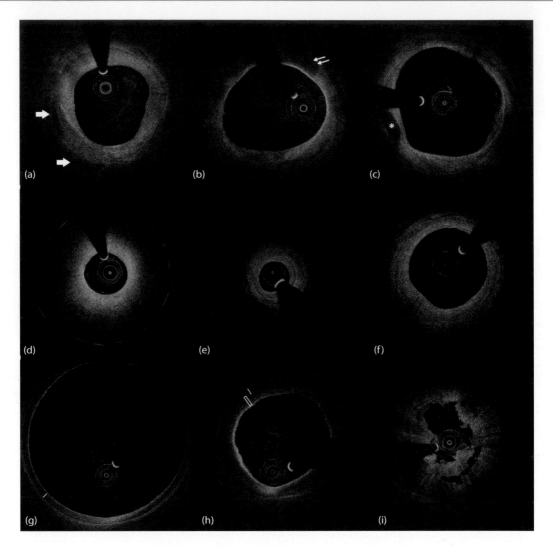

Figure 9.2 Intravascular pathologies of the lower extremity identified by OCT. (a) Fibrotic plaque with high signal (bright) and low attenuation (deep penetration); underlying calcium deposits (broad arrows) are noted as well. (b) Lipid-rich plaques (narrow arrows) are low signal lesions (dark) with irregular borders and high attenuation (poor tissue penetration). (c) Calcified plaques (asterisk) are also low signal lesions, but are characterized by discrete borders and can cause some protrusion of the arterial wall into the intraluminal space. These are low-attenuation lesions, which permits visualization of tissue below the calcium. (d) Diffuse NIH in a previously stented lesion; stent struts are well expanded. (e) Neointimal fibrotic hyperplasia of a distal arterial target, the posterior tibial artery in a patient with previous saphenous venous femoral–tibial graft. (f) A widely patent venous graft is present proximal to the venous–tibial anastomosis. Intravascular imaging of the EIA proximal to (g) and at (h), the level of arterial vasospasm. There is no evidence of atherosclerosis at the level of vasospasm, although there is an increase in the thickness of both the tunica media (single line) and intima (rectangle). Distal to the segment of the vasospasm, the thickness of the medial and intimal layers returns to baseline and is similar to that of the proximal segment (not shown). (i) White thrombus, which is signal-rich, but unlike red thrombus, it has low attenuation with low-backscattering projections.

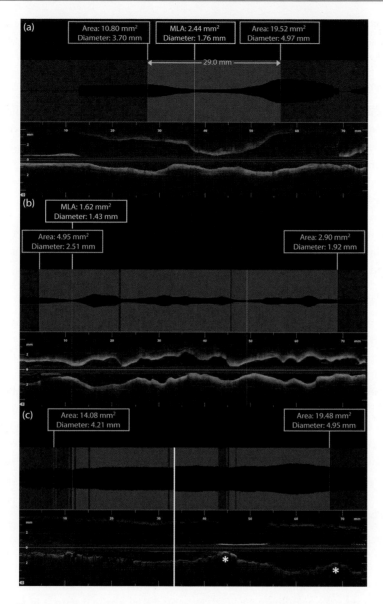

Figure 9.3 Lumen profile and axial imaging along the catheter plane can provide a gestalt of the severity of disease, but also guide therapeutic intervention by way of reference vessel diameter and length of target lesion. (a) In this patient with a focal SFA stenosis, the minimal luminal area is measured to be 2.44 mm², with a reference vessel diameter distally of 3.70 mm and proximally of 4.97 mm. The total lesion length is measured to be 29.0 mm. (b) The lumen profile and axial imaging illustrate the widespread ISR in this patient with recurrent claudication after prior SFA stenting. (c) Poststent placement evaluation of the SFA, with a distal Supera stent (left of white line) and an overlapping Absolute Pro SE stent (right of white line). The white line marks the overlapped region, with asterisks highlighting the malapposed portions of the Absolute Pro SE stent. MLA, minimum lumen area.

a subtotally occlusive lesion consistent with NIH of the posterior tibial artery, beyond the distal anastomosis. OCT confirms the presence of a severe fibrotic stenosis in the native artery (Figure 9.2e); the anastomosis and vein graft are widely patent (Figure 9.2f).

9.4.1.5 Vasospasm: case 5

A 42-year-old woman with a smoking history but otherwise unremarkable prior medical history presents after cardiac arrest while playing golf. Upon evaluation by the emergency medical services, she is found to have polymorphic ventricular tachycardia. Transient anterior stent thrombosis (ST)–segment elevation is present on electrocardiogram soon after her arrival at the hospital. She undergoes emergent coronary angiogram, showing proximal left anterior descending stenosis with near-complete resolution with injection of intracoronary nitroglycerin.

At the conclusion of the case, the peripheral angiogram shows focal stenosis of the external iliac artery (EIA), with modest improvement following intra-arterial nitroglycerin. OCT of the EIA reveals no evidence of atherosclerotic plaque, although within the spasmodic region, there is evidence of increased thickness of both the intimal and medial layers (Figure 9.2g and h).[28]

9.4.1.6 Thrombus: case 6

A 55-year-old man with a history of myocardial infarction requiring coronary stenting 12 years ago presents with right lower extremity claudication consistent with Rutherford Stage 3 symptoms. A selective right peripheral angiogram shows focal midvessel occlusion with two-vessel runoff. On OCT, a heavy burden of white thrombus is noted (Figure 9.2i).

The differentiation between red and white thrombus by use of OCT characterization compared with cadaveric histology has previously been described in the coronary literature.[29] Red thrombus, composed of primarily red blood cells, is signal-rich superficially but has low penetration, resulting in high-backscattering protrusions with signal-free shadowing.[17,29–31] On the other hand, white thrombus is composed of platelets and white blood cells. On OCT, it is also signal-rich but with lower attenuation with low-backscattering protrusions.[17,29–31]

9.4.2 Assessment of interventional techniques

9.4.2.1 Angioplasty

9.4.2.1.1 Balloon angioplasty: back to case 1

Percutaneous transluminal angioplasty (PTA) is performed with a 4.0 × 40 mm focal force balloon. A post-intervention angiogram and concomitant OCT show satisfactory luminal gain. On OCT, a Grade I focal dissection is noted (Figure 9.4a).

9.4.2.1.2 Cutting balloon: back to case 4

Cutting balloon angioplasty is performed of the posterior tibial artery lesion using a 2.5 × 10 mm focal force balloon. Postinflation angiography demonstrates contrast flow into the medial plantar artery. However, OCT shows diffuse residual debris and an irregular endothelial surface after plaque fracture (Figure 9.4b). These findings precipitate additional prolonged inflation PTA using a 3.0 × 20 mm balloon. The final angiography shows improved runoff without remnant pathology. Postintervention OCT imaging shows marked luminal gain with clear demonstration of the cutting balloon fracture clefts within the lesion (Figure 9.4c).

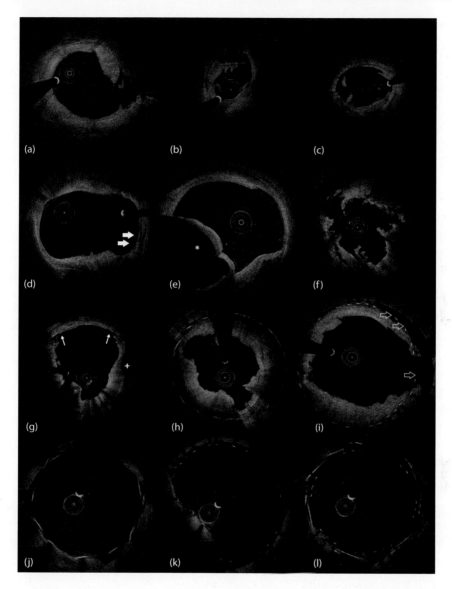

Figure 9.4 OCT-guided interventional therapies in the lower extremity. (a) Focal force balloon angioplasty of a focal SFA lesion, creating a Grade I focal dissection. Use of a cutting balloon (b), followed by prolonged balloon inflation with a traditional angioplasty catheter (c) in a posterior tibial artery; note the presence of residual cutting balloon fracture clefts after PTA in the latter depiction. In a patient with restenosis after prior PTA of the SFA, directional atherectomy is performed with disruption of the intimal and medial layers (d, broad arrows), although only modest luminal gain. Subsequent PTA resulted in a spiral dissection (e), with an associated false lumen (asterisk) necessitating stenting. A patient with subtotal proximal SFA occlusion undergoes orbital atherectomy with diffuse plaque disruption (f), followed by PTA (g) resulting in a non-flow-limiting dissection (narrow arrows) with residual calcium (plus sign). Laser atherectomy is performed in a patient with severe and diffuse ISR (h), followed by high-pressure PTA with notable dissection (hollow arrows) behind prior stent struts (i). A well-expanded and well-apposed stent (j) compared with a well-expanded but malapposed stent (k). The overlapped segment of the two stents (l), with the Supera stent forming the outer layer and the Absolute Pro SE the inner layer, illustrates the dependence of radial forces on stent design.

9.4.2.2 Atherectomy

9.4.2.2.1 Directional atherectomy: back to case 1

The patient returns with recurrence of claudication symptoms approximately 4 months following her index procedure. A peripheral angiogram reveals 95% restenosis in the prior angioplasty site. OCT demonstrates fibrosis along with lipid-rich and calcific plaques.

Directional atherectomy (Turbohawk, Covidien, Mansfield, Massachusetts) is advanced and multiple passes are made. Repeat angiogram with OCT shows residual 40% stenosis (Figure 9.4d). PTA is performed at this time, complicated by spiral dissection on OCT (Figure 9.4e). Two overlapping self-expanding nitinol stents are placed, with final OCT showing well-expanded and well-apposed stents without residual dissection.

9.4.2.2.2 Orbital atherectomy: back to case 2

The subtotal occlusion is crossed with a guidewire and orbital atherectomy is applied (Diamondback, Cardiovascular Systems Inc., St. Paul, Minnesota). The resultant OCT shows diffuse plaque disruption (Figure 9.4f). Dilation using a 5.0 × 100 mm balloon yields a residual 50% stenosis, and subsequent dilation with a 6.0 × 100 mm balloon results in a non-flow-limiting dissection and residual calcium apparent on OCT (Figure 9.4g). Two overlapping self-expanding nitinol stents are placed without residual stenosis or dissection, and the two-vessel runoff via the anterior and posterior tibial arteries is dramatically improved.

Laser atherectomy: Back to Case 3. With extensive NIH, debulking is necessary for procedural success. Three passes are made by a laser atherectomy catheter at progressively escalating fluency and repetition rates, with modest resultant luminal gain (Figure 9.4h). Further plaque modification is performed using a 6.0 × 100 mm cutting balloon. OCT demonstrates significantly improved luminal gain, although complicated by a proximal dissection flap evident behind the stent struts (Figure 9.4i). To further decrease the recurrence of ISR, a 6.0 × 100 mm drug-coated balloon is used for final dilation.

9.4.2.3 Stent

9.4.2.3.1 Malapposition: back to case 2

The patient returns 2 months later for intervention on his left lower extremity. On angiography, a long-segment chronic total occlusion (CTO) is noted of the left SFA, with reconstitution via profunda femoral artery collaterals near Hunter's canal. The CTO is successfully crossed, and after confirmation of intraluminal positioning, progressive predilation is performed.

A self-expanding 5.0 × 120 mm Supera stent (Abbott Vascular, Santa Clara, California) is placed in the distal SFA, followed by two overlapping 6.0 × 100 mm Absolute Pro stents (Abbott Vascular). After post-dilation, final OCT pullback shows a well-expanded and well-apposed Supera stent (Figure 9.4j), while the Absolute Pro stent (Figure 9.4k) is malapposed despite adequate expansion; this is outlined in the luminal profile (Figure 9.3c). The overlapping section of the two stents highlights how differences in stent design can have an impact on the radial forces generated *in vivo* (Figure 9.4l).[32,33]

9.5 FUTURE DIRECTIONS

OCT has been applied in the peripheral vasculature in largely experimental applications. Despite lacking Food and Drug Administration (FDA) approval specifically for this indication, there does appear to be an emerging role for OCT imaging in peripheral vascular arterial disease assessment. Ongoing advancements in OCT technology have rendered its adjunctive use in extracoronary procedures increasingly accessible, with applications in not only the peripheral vascular system but also the renal and carotid arteries.[16,34–36] Prior difficulties (e.g., vessel size, lesion length, and need for occlusive imaging) that had limited its use in the extracoronary vasculature no longer present a barrier to the application of OCT in the peripheral vasculature. Its superior imaging quality compared with IVUS may offer insights into the diagnosis and treatment of PAD, and may supplant IVUS as the intravascular imaging modality of choice in the future.

REFERENCES

1. Lin JS et al. *The Ankle Brachial Index for Peripheral Artery Disease Screening and Cardiovascular Disease Prediction in Asymptomatic Adults: A Systematic Evidence Review for the US Preventive Services Task Force*. Rockville, MD: Agency for Healthcare Research and Quality, 2013.
2. Cassar K. Peripheral arterial disease. *BMJ Clinical Evidence* 2011. Available at http://clinicalevidence.bmj.com/x/systematic-review/0211/overview.html.
3. Norgren L et al. Inter-society consensus for the management of peripheral arterial disease (TASC II). *Journal of Vascular Surgery* 2007;45(Suppl S):S5–67.
4. Fogarty TJ et al. A method for extraction of arterial emboli and thrombi. *Surgery, Gynecology & Obstetrics* 1963;116:241–4.
5. Scoccianti M et al. Intravascular ultrasound guidance for peripheral vascular interventions. *Journal of Endovascular Surgery* 1994;1:71–80.
6. Fogarty TJ, Cranley JJ. Catheter technic for arterial embolectomy. *Annals of Surgery* 1965;161:325–30.
7. Payne MM. Charles Theodore Dotter. The father of intervention. *Texas Heart Institute Journal* 2001;28:28–38.
8. Friedman SG. Charles Dotter and the fiftieth anniversary of endovascular surgery. *Journal of Vascular Surgery* 2015;61:556–8.
9. Lee JT et al. Applications of intravascular ultrasound in the treatment of peripheral occlusive disease. *Seminars in Vascular Surgery* 2006;19:139–44.
10. Cronenwett JL, Johnston KW. *Rutherford's Vascular Surgery*. New York: Elsevier Health Sciences, 2014.
11. Moscucci M. *Grossman & Baim's Cardiac Catheterization, Angiography, and Intervention*. Philadelphia: Wolters Kluwer Health, 2013.
12. Secco GG et al. Optical coherence tomography guidance during peripheral vascular intervention. *Cardiovascular and Interventional Radiology* 2015;38:768–72.
13. Farooq MU et al. The role of optical coherence tomography in vascular medicine. *Vascular Medicine* 2009;14:63–71.
14. Diethrich EB et al. Virtual histology and color flow intravascular ultrasound in peripheral interventions. *Seminars in Vascular Surgery* 2006;19:155–62.
15. Bezerra HG et al. Optical coherence tomography versus intravascular ultrasound to evaluate coronary artery disease and percutaneous coronary intervention. *JACC Cardiovascular Interventions* 2013;6:228–36.
16. Negi SI, Rosales O. The role of intravascular optical coherence tomography in peripheral percutaneous interventions. *Journal of Invasive Cardiology* 2013;25:E51–3.
17. Bezerra HG et al. Intracoronary optical coherence tomography: A comprehensive review: Clinical and research applications. *JACC Cardiovascular Interventions* 2009;2:1035–46.
18. Stefano GT et al. Imaging a spiral dissection of the superficial femoral artery in high resolution with optical coherence tomography—Seeing is believing. *Catheterization and Cardiovascular Interventions* 2013;81:568–72.
19. Eberhardt KM et al. Prospective evaluation of optical coherence tomography in lower limb arteries compared with intravascular ultrasound. *Journal of Vascular and Interventional Radiology* 2013;24:1499–508.
20. Kendrick D et al. PS78. The OPTIMISE Trial: Intravascular optical coherence tomography in lower extremity arteries. *Journal of Vascular Surgery* 59:53S–4S.
21. Karnabatidis D et al. Frequency-domain intravascular optical coherence tomography of the femoropopliteal artery. *Cardiovascular and Interventional Radiology* 2011;34:1172–81.
22. Paraskevopoulos I et al. Evaluation of below-the-knee drug-eluting stents with frequency-domain optical coherence tomography: Neointimal hyperplasia and neoatherosclerosis. *Journal of Endovascular Therapy* 2013;20:80–93.
23. Pomposelli F. Arterial imaging in patients with lower extremity ischemia and diabetes mellitus. *Journal of Vascular Surgery* 2010;52:81S–91S.

24. Abdulghaffar W et al. Role of carbon dioxide angiography in management of below knee arterial lesions. *Egyptian Journal of Radiology and Nuclear Medicine* 2012;43:549–54.

25. Gonzalo N et al. Optical coherence tomography patterns of stent restenosis. *American Heart Journal* 2009;158:284–93.

26. Vergallo R et al. Correlation between degree of neointimal hyperplasia and incidence and characteristics of neoatherosclerosis as assessed by optical coherence tomography. *American Journal of Cardiology* 2013;112:1315–21.

27. Kim JS et al. Long-term outcomes of neointimal hyperplasia without neoatherosclerosis after drug-eluting stent implantation. *JACC Cardiovascular Imaging* 2014;7:788–95.

28. Basuray A et al. A shocking front nine: Cardiac arrest on the golf course. *Circulation* 2012;126:2526–32.

29. Kume T et al. Assessment of coronary arterial thrombus by optical coherence tomography. *American Journal of Cardiology* 2006;97:1713–7.

30. Kume T et al. Images in cardiovascular medicine. Fibrin clot visualized by optical coherence tomography. *Circulation* 2008;118:426–7.

31. Tearney GJ et al. Consensus standards for acquisition, measurement, and reporting of intravascular optical coherence tomography studies: A report from the International Working Group for Intravascular Optical Coherence Tomography Standardization and Validation. *Journal of the American College of Cardiology* 2012;59:1058–72.

32. Abbott Vascular. Supera Peripheral Stent System: Instructions for use. Santa Clara, CA: Abbott Vascular, 2014.

33. Gates L, Indes J. New treatment of iliac artery disease: Focus on the Absolute Pro® Vascular Self-Expanding Stent System. *Medical Devices (Auckland, NZ)* 2013;6:147–50.

34. Bastante T, Alfonso F. Insights of optical coherence tomography in renal artery fibromuscular dysplasia in a patient with spontaneous coronary artery dissection. *Arquivos Brasileiros de Cardiologia* 2014;103:e18.

35. Templin C et al. Vascular lesions induced by renal nerve ablation as assessed by optical coherence tomography: Pre- and post-procedural comparison with the Simplicity catheter system and the EnligHTN multi-electrode renal denervation catheter. *European Heart Journal* 2013;34:2141–8, 2148b.

36. Yoshimura S et al. OCT of human carotid arterial plaques. *JACC Cardiovascular Imaging* 2011;4:432–6.

Chapter 10

Optical coherence tomography for the assessment of bioresorbable vascular scaffolds

Yohei Ohno, Alessio La Manna, and Corrado Tamburino

10.1 INTRODUCTION

Bioresorbable vascular scaffolds (BVSs) (Abbott Vascular, Redwood City, California) have been proposed as the fourth revolution in percutaneous coronary intervention (PCI).[1] These novel coronary devices have been recently introduced in the clinical practice as an alternative to the conventional metallic drug-eluting stent (DES) for the percutaneous treatment of coronary artery disease. The rationale of BVS use is based on the concept of so-called "vascular restoration therapy," which is based on the temporary scaffolding provided by the bioresorbable prosthesis, as opposed to the permanent caging determined by DES implantation. The benefits of BVS treatment should consist of the transient scaffolding effect that is followed by progressive bioresorption of the scaffold, and finally the restoration of the normal coronary anatomy and vasoreactivity, with the subsequent elimination of the risk of late stent thrombosis due to the absence of persistent strut malapposition and chronically uncovered struts, and on the other hand, the late lumen gain secondary to expansive remodeling and plaque regression that may reduce the risk of restenosis and delay disease progression. Other benefits arising from BVS therapy include the possibility for future surgical revascularization and the potential for the noninvasive imaging of coronary arteries with multislice computed tomography and magnetic resonance. Currently available preliminary data show that BVSs could be a safe and effective alternative to second-generation DESs in selected patients with stable coronary lesions of mild to moderate complexity.[2] Several studies are ongoing and will shortly provide a larger amount of data on the safety and efficacy of BVSs in more complex and higher-risk patient populations.

Regarding the design, the BVS platform is made of three different components: (1) poly-L-lactide (PLLA), a semicrystalline fully metabolized polymer that constitutes the scaffold backbone providing the mechanical properties (i.e., radial strength) of the prosthesis; (2) the bioresorbable coating, which is made of poly-D,L-lactide (PDLLA), an amorphous fully metabolized polymer that is responsible for the drug release; and (3) the antiproliferative drug everolimus, which is embedded in the PDLLA with the same dose density and release rate as the Xience V DES. This technical specification is important since the building material of the BVS has an impact on its mechanical properties and, consequently, on the management of the PCI when BVS implantation is planned.

10.2   OPTICAL COHERENCE TOMOGRAPHY ASSESSMENT BEFORE BVS IMPLANTATION

Since the BVS platform is made of polymer, its design and mechanical properties clearly differ from those of metallic DESs. First, the template thickness is around 150 μm, that is, about two times thicker than that of corresponding DESs (81 μm, Xience V), making the BVS profile larger than that of second-generation DESs, and thus affecting device deliverability. Second, there is a trend toward a higher acute scaffold recoil compared with that of Xience V, partly dependent on plaque morphology (i.e., calcium deposits),[3] with a significant discrepancy between acute BVS expansion and compliance chart information (Figure 10.1).[4] Third, the possibility of overexpanding the BVS is quite limited compared with metallic DESs because beyond the 0.5 mm expansion limit, there is an actual risk for fracture (Figure 10.2).[5] Because of these mechanical characteristics of BVSs, lesion preparation and proper vessel sizing are of paramount importance in order to accomplish an adequate delivery of the scaffold. Optical coherence tomography (OCT) has become the gold standard for the invasive assessment of plaque morphology and strut apposition compared with intravascular ultrasound (IVUS).[6] In particular, OCT can better delineate the presence and extent of vessel calcification that may hamper the deliverability and adequate expansion of BVSs because of scaffold recoil, and it may serve as a guide for lesion preparation, suggesting the use of debulking devices like rotational aterectomy or excimer laser angioplasty and/or scoring balloons in order to achieve a satisfactory vessel expansion before BVS delivery. Indeed, residual calcium arc or calcium nodules may limit the expansion of BVSs and be predictive of strut malapposition, suggesting the alternative use of metallic DESs (Figure 10.3). OCT can guide each step of lesion preparation from the baseline assessment of plaque morphology to the evaluation of the effect of debulking procedures in order to finally proceed to BVS deployment. Importantly, this could be particularly relevant in the case of bifurcation lesion treatment[7] because access to the side branches after BVS implantation may become difficult, and the OCT assessment of plaque distribution at the bifurcation site before scaffolding may influence the lesion preparation strategy.

Another important technical feature of BVSs is the limited possibility to overexpand the scaffold for the risk of frame fracture.[5] Currently available metallic DESs offer a wide range of overexpansion since most of them can be dilated up to 1.5 mm over the specified diameter, making them adaptable to vessel segments of varying sizes.[8] Due to the narrow range of BVS overexpansion, proper vessel sizing of the target vessel is more important than in the case of DESs and becomes key in order to achieve adequate strut apposition. OCT is the most accurate imaging method to assess vessel size compared with IVUS[9] and quantitative coronary angiography (QCA)[10] because of the higher spatial resolution. OCT-based measurement of reference

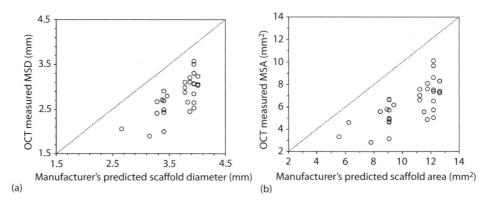

(a)   (b)

Figure 10.1 (a) Scatter plot of the predicted and actual minimum scaffold diameters. (b) Similar graph of predicted and actual minimum scaffold areas.

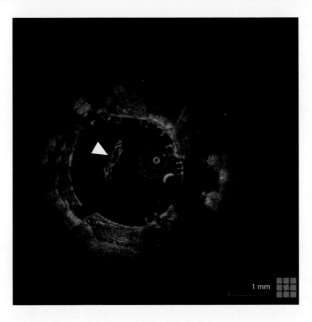

Figure 10.2 Representative image of BVS fracture in severely calcified plaque. Isolated struts (white arrowhead) are located more or less at the center of the vessel without obvious connection to other surrounding struts in 2D OCT, which confirms the diagnosis of acute strut fracture.

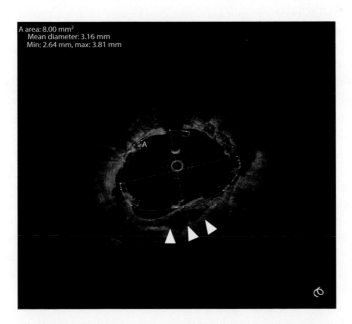

Figure 10.3 Representative image of BVS implantation in calcified plaque. BVS expansion is limited in the direction of calcified plaque (white arrowheads), demonstrating uneven expansion with malapposed BVS struts.

vessel diameter allows us to choose the correct BVS diameter, reducing the risk of incomplete scaffold apposition, potentially triggering scaffold thrombosis, and consequently avoiding the need for aggressive BVS overexpansion that may lead to frame fracture and in turn itself be the cause of scaffold thrombosis and restenosis due to strut protrusion and loss in radial strength. Furthermore, OCT can provide a precise estimation of lesion length, enabling a complete plaque sealing by BVSs, and thus potentially improving both the short-term result through the reduction of the risk of edge dissection and the long-term outcome through the BVS-mediated vessel reparative process, which could be particularly important in the case of residual vulnerable plaque, as it is currently being investigated.

10.3   OPTICAL COHERENCE TOMOGRAPHY ASSESSMENT AFTER BVS IMPLANTATION

After BVS implantation, there are several things that should be carefully observed with OCT. First, assessing the expansion and apposition of BVS struts is of importance. Possible scaffold disruption or fracture should also be identified, if any. The diagnosis of acute strut fracture resulting from balloon overdilation or late structural strut discontinuity can be established if two struts overhang each other in the same angular sector of the lumen perimeter, with or without malapposition, or if isolated struts are located more or less at the center of the vessel without obvious connection to other surrounding struts in two-dimensional (2D) OCT (Figure 10.2).[11] For confirmation of the diagnosis, it is helpful to perform three-dimensional (3D) OCT reconstruction of the disrupted strut. In a previous study, we demonstrated that a BVS almost always underexpands compared with the predicted area (Figure 10.1), and it is prominent when underlying plaques are calcified.[4] Early and midterm outcomes from the European multicenter GHOST-EU registry[12] have demonstrated a relatively high incidence of scaffold thrombosis (2.1% at 6 months). Aside from the fact that this study included patients who were treated under an early learning curve, considering that approximately 70% of scaffold thrombosis cases occurred within 30 days, and only 15% of cases were treated under intravascular imaging (i.e., IVUS or OCT) guidance, one could easily imagine that this was partially related to the procedure, i.e., possible underexpansion or malapposition. Therefore, OCT-guided postdilation after BVS implantation to achieve good expansion without leaving malapposition is strongly recommended using a noncompliant balloon. At baseline, the scaffold area is measured by joining the middle point of the black core abluminal side of the apposed struts (Figure 10.4a) or the abluminal edge of the frame borders of malapposed struts (Figure 10.4b).

Second, in the case of multiple BVS implantation for one lesion, the overlapped segment has to be assessed carefully (Figure 10.5a). There are potential concerns of using BVSs in an overlap fashion: (1) Thick struts might lead to flow disruption and its potential adverse consequences (i.e., scaffold thrombosis), which is especially relevant in small vessels since two scaffold layers can easily occupy the vessel lumen. (2) Real-world clinical data regarding the acute interaction between the two scaffold layers and the artery wall, as well as the vascular response over time, are still lacking. (3) Bifurcation techniques, such as the crush technique with three partial layers of scaffold (Figure 10.5b), might magnify the concerns mentioned here. The difficult part of making a good overlap (i.e., minimum overlap or completely adjacent implantation without overlapping) is that (1) the polymeric scaffold is not visible under fluoro, and (2) the platinum markers at both ends are not the real "ends" of the scaffolds, i.e., the struts exist both distal to the distal platinum marker and proximal to the proximal platinum marker, depending on the size of the BVS.

Third, similarly with metallic DESs, edge dissection can occur after BVS implantation, which might lead to early or late BVS failure. Therefore, careful observation is necessary in order to assess the extent and depth of the edge dissection, which might be helpful to decide whether to implant another BVS.

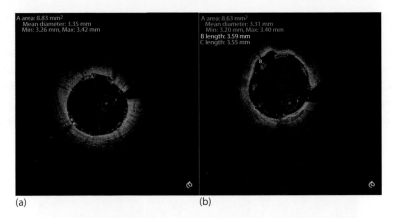

Figure 10.4 Measurement of the scaffold area. The scaffold area is measured by joining the middle point of the black core abluminal side of the apposed struts (a) or the abluminal edge of the frame borders of the malapposed struts (b).

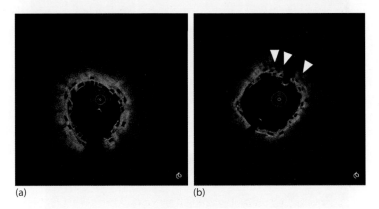

Figure 10.5 (a) Overlapped segments of BVS. (b) Three partial layers of scaffold (white arrowheads) are shown after BVS implantation in a bifurcation lesion with the crush technique.

Fourth, the longitudinal integrity of the BVS should be assessed. It has been shown that in particular settings (i.e., hard calcified plaque and high implantation pressure), BVSs can elongate longitudinally. The potential procedural implications of BVS elongation could be as follows: (1) missing adequate position in ostial lesions (i.e., extending the scaffold to the left main without the intention to do so), (2) longer than predicted overlapping segments, and (3) landing the stent in a diseased segment (i.e., adjacent to the normal target landing zone).

10.4 OPTICAL COHERENCE TOMOGRAPHY ASSESSMENT FOR BVS FOLLOW-UP

Previous studies have shown that BVS struts start to be covered with neointima 6–9 months after implantation. The thickness of the coverage can be measured in every strut between the abluminal site of the strut core and the lumen. Since the strut thickness is 150 μm, the strut is considered covered whenever the thickness of the coverage is above this threshold value. This method may slightly underestimate the thickness of the coverage because it does not take into account changes in the size of the strut core over time. Consequently, the percentage of uncovered struts may be slightly overestimated. The lumen and scaffold contours are obtained with a semiautomated detection algorithm available in many offline software packages, and additional manual corrections are performed if necessary. At follow-up, the luminal area is drawn by semiautomatic detection, following the endoluminal contour of the neointima between and on top of the apposed struts. For malapposed struts, the endoluminal contour of the vessel wall behind the malapposed struts is used. The back (abluminal) side of the central black core is used to delimit the scaffold area. Representative cases of bifurcation using two BVSs and chronic total occlusion treated with multiple BVSs are shown in Figures 10.6 and 10.7.

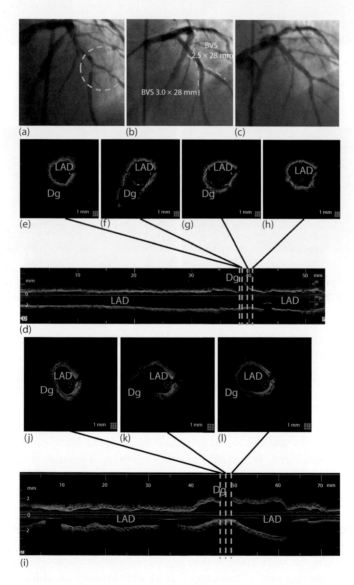

Figure 10.6 Percutaneous coronary intervention for bifurcation lesion using two BVSs. Coronary angiography at baseline (a), after PCI (b), and at the 2-year follow-up (c). (d–h) OCT images after BVS implantation. (f) Well-apposed struts in the side branch (Dg) ostium and main branch (LAD) are observed. (g) Minimally overlapped struts that are slightly malapposed are observed. (i–l) OCT images at the 2-year follow-up. All struts at the bifurcation are well covered with neointima.

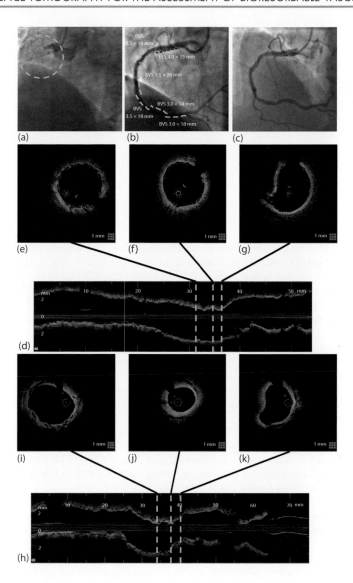

Figure 10.7 Percutaneous coronary intervention for chronic total occlusion lesion treated with multiple BVSs. Coronary angiography at baseline (a), after PCI (b), and at the 1-year follow-up (c). (d–g) OCT images after BVS implantation. Well-apposed struts in both overlapped (d) and nonoverlapped (e) segments. (f) Minimum incomplete apposition in calcified plaque is observed. (h–k) OCT images at the 1-year follow-up. No scaffold recoil is observed in both overlapped (i) and nonoverlapped (j) segments. (j) Diffuse neointimal proliferation is shown with a minimal lumen area of 3.5 mm^2. (k) The previous minimally malapposed segment is covered with neointima.

The ABSORB II trial recently showed comparable 1-year composite secondary clinical outcomes of BVSs compared with second-generation everolimus-eluting stents, with 5% of patients treated with BVSs experiencing target lesion failure (TLF) at 1 year.[13] In a large real-world registry (n = 1189) including more complex clinical and angiographic characteristics than those represented in the ABSORB II trial, the rate of TLF was 4.4% at 6 months.[12] It is of particular importance to understand the underlying mechanism of BVS failure by using OCT in order to select the appropriate intervention. We have recently reported a series of BVS failure and showed that geographical misses resulting in abnormal edge vascular response and scaffold underexpansion were the most prevalent causes identified.[14] However, the optimal management for BVS failure is still not yet established since at the time of the event the scaffold has generally lost part of its mechanical properties and simple dilation may disrupt the struts with uncertain outcomes.[15]

DISCLOSURES

All authors have no relationships relevant to the contents of this chapter to disclose.

REFERENCES

1. Ormiston JA, Serruys PW. Bioabsorbable coronary stents. *Circulation Cardiovascular Interventions* 2009;2:255–60.
2. Abizaid A, Costa JR, Jr., Bartorelli AL, Whitbourn R, van Geuns RJ, Chevalier B, Patel T, Seth A, Stuteville M, Dorange C, Cheong WF, Sudhir K and Serruys PW. The ABSORB EXTEND study: Preliminary report of the twelve-month clinical outcomes in the first 512 patients enrolled. *EuroIntervention* 2015;10:1396–401.
3. Brown AJ, McCormick LM, Braganza DM, Bennett MR, Hoole SP and West NE. Expansion and malapposition characteristics after bioresorbable vascular scaffold implantation. *Catheterization and Cardiovascular Interventions* 2014;84:37–45.
4. Attizzani GF, Ohno Y, Capodanno D, Francaviglia B, Grasso C, Sgroi C, Wang W, Fujino Y, Ganocy SJ, Longo G, Tamburino CI, Di Salvo M, La Manna A, Capranzano P and Tamburino C. New insights on acute expansion and longitudinal elongation of bioresorbable vascular scaffolds in vivo and at bench test: A note of caution on reliance to compliance charts and nominal length. *Catheterization and Cardiovascular Interventions* 2015;85:E99–107.
5. Ormiston JA, De Vroey F, Serruys PW and Webster MW. Bioresorbable polymeric vascular scaffolds: A cautionary tale. *Circulation Cardiovascular Interventions* 2011;4:535–8.
6. Prati F, Guagliumi G, Mintz GS, Costa M, Regar E, Akasaka T, Barlis P, Tearney GJ, Jang IK, Arbustini E, Bezerra HG, Ozaki Y, Bruining N, Dudek D, Radu M, Erglis A, Motreff P, Alfonso F, Toutouzas K, Gonzalo N, Tamburino C, Adriaenssens T, Pinto F, Serruys PW, Di Mario C and Expert's OCTRD. Expert review document part 2: Methodology, terminology and clinical applications of optical coherence tomography for the assessment of interventional procedures. *European Heart Journal* 2012;33:2513–20.
7. Attizzani GF, Ohno Y, Capranzano P, La Manna A, Francaviglia B, Grasso C, Sgroi C, Tamburino C, Longo G, Fujino Y, Capodanno D and Tamburino C. Initial experience of percutaneous coronary intervention in bifurcations with bioresorbable vascular scaffolds using different techniques—Insights from optical coherence tomography. *International Journal of Cardiology* 2013;170:e33–5.
8. Foin N, Sen S, Allegria E, Petraco R, Nijjer S, Francis DP, Di Mario C and Davies JE. Maximal expansion capacity with current DES platforms: A critical factor for stent selection in the treatment of left main bifurcations? *EuroIntervention* 2013;8:1315–25.
9. Bezerra HG, Costa MA, Guagliumi G, Rollins AM and Simon DI. Intracoronary optical coherence tomography: A comprehensive review clinical and research applications. *JACC Cardiovascular Interventions* 2009;2:1035–46.
10. Dahm JB, van Buuren F. Low resolution limits and inaccurate algorithms decrease significantly the value of late loss in current drug-eluting stent trials. *International Journal of Vascular Medicine* 2012;2012:417250.
11. Garcia-Garcia HM, Serruys PW, Campos CM, Muramatsu T, Nakatani S, Zhang YJ, Onuma Y and Stone GW. Assessing bioresorbable coronary devices: Methods and parameters. *JACC Cardiovascular Imaging* 2014;7:1130–48.
12. Capodanno D, Gori T, Nef H, Latib A, Mehilli J, Lesiak M, Caramanno G, Naber C, Di Mario C, Colombo A, Capranzano P, Wiebe J, Araszkiewicz A, Geraci S, Pyxaras S, Mattesini A, Naganuma T, Munzel T and Tamburino C. Percutaneous coronary intervention with everolimus-eluting bioresorbable vascular scaffolds in routine clinical practice: Early and midterm outcomes from the European multicentre GHOST-EU registry. *EuroIntervention* 2015;10:1144–53.

13. Serruys PW, Chevalier B, Dudek D, Cequier A, Carrie D, Iniguez A, Dominici M, van der Schaaf RJ, Haude M, Wasungu L, Veldhof S, Peng L, Staehr P, Grundeken MJ, Ishibashi Y, Garcia-Garcia HM and Onuma Y. A bioresorbable everolimus-eluting scaffold versus a metallic everolimus-eluting stent for ischaemic heart disease caused by de-novo native coronary artery lesions (ABSORB II): An interim 1-year analysis of clinical and procedural secondary outcomes from a randomised controlled trial. *Lancet* 2015;385:43–54.
14. Longo G, Granata F, Capodanno D, Ohno Y, Tamburino CI, Capranzano P, La Manna A, Francaviglia B, Gargiulo G and Tamburino C. Anatomical features and management of bioresorbable vascular scaffolds failure: A case series from the GHOST registry. *Catheterization and Cardiovascular Interventions* 2015;85:1150–61.
15. Ohno Y, Mangiameli A, Attizzani GF, Capodanno D and Tamburino C. Optical coherence tomography assessment of late intra-scaffold dissection: A new challenge of bioresorbable scaffolds. *JACC Cardiovascular Interventions* 2015;8:e11–2.

Chapter 11

ILUMIEN OPTIS Mobile and OPTIS Integrated Technology Overview

Tsung-Han Tsai and Desmond Adler

11.1 PLATFORM OVERVIEW

The ILUMIEN™ OPTIS™ Mobile System and OPTIS Integrated System are the second- and third-generation, respectively, percutaneous coronary intervention (PCI) optimization platforms developed by St. Jude Medical, Inc. that have both leading-edge intravascular optical coherence tomography (OCT) imaging technology and fractional flow reserve (FFR) technology.[1,2] OCT is an imaging modality that uses fiber-optic technology and optical imaging catheters that emit near-infrared light to produce high-resolution, real-time images. The frequency and bandwidth characteristics of the near-infrared light used in these systems result in image resolution superior to that of typical medical ultrasound images.

The FFR is the ratio of the distal coronary arterial pressure to the aortic pressure, measured during hyperemia. It provides the maximal blood flow in the presence of a stenosis as a fraction of the achievable blood flow that would exist in the hypothetical situation that the stenosis was not present. The physician may use the FFR parameter, along with knowledge of patient history, medical expertise, and clinical judgment, to determine if therapeutic intervention is indicated. This functionality is achieved when the PCI Optimization System is used in conjunction with the manufacturer's wireless distal intracoronary pressure transducer and a proximal aortic pressure transducer.

The ILUMIEN OPTIS Mobile System is a mobile cart-based system using state-of-the-art OCT technology, and can offer real-time three-dimensional (3D) vessel reconstruction and stent planning tools for optimal PCI decision making. The OPTIS Integrated System builds on the functionality of the ILUMIEN OPTIS system, but is installed into the catheter lab so that OCT and the FFR are immediately available without the need to find, connect, position, and power-on a mobile console. The system allows either the sterile operator or nonsterile operator to control system functions during image and FFR acquisition and review, and to view the OCT and FFR images on the main catheter lab monitor boom. In addition, the OPTIS Integrated System incorporates angio coregistration (ACR), which allows the user to visualize the position of OCT image data on angiography images, tightening the linkage between anatomical assessment with OCT and subsequent therapeutic actions.

11.1.1 FD-OCT operating principles

OCT originated from a technique known as low-coherence interferometry, which uses a Michelson interferometer with a broadband light source.[3–5] In the traditional time-domain OCT (TD-OCT) configuration, the reference arm of the interferometer has a mechanical scanning reference path delay that is translated over the desired imaging depth. Optical interference between the light from the sample and reference arms occurs only when the optical delays match and the backscattered light intensity profile at different imaging depths (axial scans) can be measured.[6,7]

Fourier-domain OCT (FD-OCT) employs the Fourier-domain detection techniques and results in imaging speeds 10–200 times faster and a detection sensitivity 10- to 100-fold greater than traditional TD-OCT.[8–10] While TD-OCT measures the interference signal intensity at different depths, FD-OCT measures the spectrum of the interference signal without the need for mechanically changing the reference path delay. The OCT axial scan can be obtained by applying Fourier transformation on the detected spectrum.[8–10] There are two major FD-OCT techniques, including the spectral/Fourier-domain OCT (SD-OCT) and swept-source OCT (SS-OCT). SD-OCT uses a high-speed spectrometer to measure the spectrum of the OCT interference signal and has been broadly used in clinical ophthalmology because it enables ultra-high resolutions, as well as 3D imaging of retinal pathologies.[11–14] SS-OCT uses a wavelength-swept laser light source and a high-speed photodetector to measure the interference spectrum.[15–19] SS-OCT enables operation at near-infrared wavelengths of 1 and 1.3 µm, which reduces optical scattering and improves imaging depth in the biological tissues, and thus is an ideal imaging technique for most biomedical applications (Figure 11.1).[20]

11.1.2 Common system specifications

The current PCI Optimization Systems have a new high-speed OCT engine that scans at 180 frames per second (fps). Higher speed allows imaging with the new 75 mm Survey mode and 54 mm High Resolution mode to provide comprehensive visualization of intravascular structures. Table 11.1 lists the common imaging specifications of the systems.

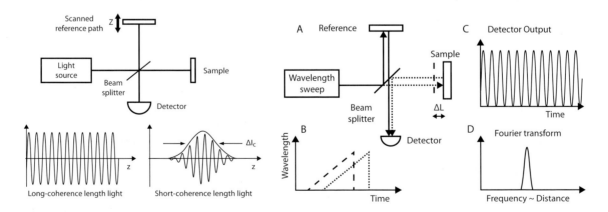

Figure 11.1 Left: TD-OCT. Right: SS-OCT.

TABLE 11.1

Imaging specifications of ILUMIEN OPTIS Mobile and Integrated Systems

Parameter	Specification
Optical Parameters: Measured at System Aperture (DOC Optical Port)	
Scanning laser source optical power	22.6 mW maximum @ 1305 ± 55 nm
	(Class 1M laser output per IEC 60825-1)
Visible laser optical power	1.45 mW maximum @ 670 nm (nominal)
	(Class 2M laser output per IEC 60825-1)
Pullback Parameters	
Pullback range	75 mm
	(If connected to a C7 Dragonfly catheter, the range is 54 mm)
Pullback speed setting	18.0 mm/s, 36.0 mm/s
	(If connected to a C7 Dragonfly catheter, the speed settings are 10.0, 20.0, and 25.0 mm/s)
General Scan Parameters	
A-Scan range in air	7.0 mm
A-Scan range in contrast	4.83 mm
Diameter measurement accuracy	7% ± 0.1 mm
Area measurement accuracy	10% ± 0.1 mm^2
Axial resolution	≤20 μm in tissue
Lateral resolution	25–60 μm
Optical sensitivity	90 dB minimum
A-Scans per second	81 kHz minimum
Frame rate	180 fps (Hz)
	(If connected to a C7 Dragonfly catheter, the frame rate is 100 fps [Hz])

11.1.3 Catheter specifications

The ILUMIEN OPTIS Mobile and OPTIS Integrated Systems are compatible with C7 Dragonfly™, Dragonfly JP/Duo, and Dragonfly OPTIS imaging catheters. The major differences between these catheters are the proximal connector design, allowing for a longer pullback range and higher-speed rotation; sheath doping for software length calibration; additional radiopaque (RO) markers to improve catheter visibility and ease deployment; and rapid exchange (RX) tip design to avoid the guidewire entering the lens area (Table 11.2). The optical performance of these catheters does not change among generations.

The Dragonfly imaging catheter consists of two main assemblies: the catheter body and the internal rotating fiber-optic imaging core. The catheter has an insertable length of 135 cm with a diameter of 2.7 Fr. It is an RX design with a "minirail" tip, having a 20 mm guidewire engagement length. The catheter has a hydrophilic coating and is designed for compatibility with 0.014 in. steerable guidewires used during coronary interventional procedures.[21–23]

Proximal to the minirail tip is the imaging area. During image acquisition, the fiber-optic core of the imaging catheter rotates and is automatically retracted within the catheter to obtain a 360° image of the artery and a continuous pullback image of an arterial segment. A luer fitting on the side arm at the proximal end of the catheter facilitates purging the central catheter lumen with 100% contrast media prior to use.

TABLE 11.2

Difference summaries of the Dragonfly imaging catheters

	C7 Dragonfly	Dragonfly JP/Duo	Dragonfly OPTIS
Torque wire	No integrated RO marker	Two integrated RO markers	Two integrated RO markers
Distal sheath	RX tip with clear window	RX tip with clear window	Dual-lumen RX tip with TiO$_2$-doped window
Proximal shaft	No shaft marker	One shaft marker at 100 cm insertion point	Two shaft markers at 90 and 100 cm insertion points
RFID	No	Yes	Yes
Maximum rotational speed	100 Hz	200 Hz	200 Hz
Maximum pullback speed	20 mm/s	40 mm/s	40 mm/s
Maximum pullback range	50 mm	75 mm	75 mm

Note: RFID, radio frequency identification.

A 3 mL syringe is required to perform the catheter purge. The catheter purge must be performed prior to imaging. The 3 mL syringe should be left attached to the side arm to allow repeated purging throughout the imaging procedure and maintain a static pressure to prevent backflow.

The C7 Dragonfly imaging catheters have two RO markers. The distal marker (minirail tip marker) is located 4 mm from the tip of the catheter, and the proximal marker (lens marker) is located 4 mm distal to the initial imaging lens position. Dragonfly JP/Duo and Dragonfly OPTIS imaging catheters have three RO markers. The most distal marker, the tip marker, is 4 mm proximal to the tip of the catheter and is affixed to the sheath. The lens marker is approximately 2 mm proximal to the lens. The most proximal marker is located 50 mm proximal to the lens marker and is used to help distinguish the imaging region. The lens and proximal markers are affixed directly to the imaging core and will move with pullback, while the tip marker will remain stationary. The imaging core can also be seen under fluoroscopy.

11.1.4 Comparison to ILUMIEN, C7xr, M3, and M2 specs

Table 11.3 lists the imaging performance of the current systems compared with earlier generations of imaging systems developed by LightLab, Inc./St. Jude Medical, Inc. The imaging speed and range are significantly increased due to the integration of the FD-OCT system and high-speed acquisition systems. The lateral scan range and catheter rotary speed increase as well due to the improvement in the imaging catheter and driver-motor and optical controller (DOC) designs. The ILUMIEN system was the first commercialized system that combines OCT imaging and wireless FFR technology to provide both anatomical and physiological information and further improve the diagnostic therapy and optimize PCI. The OC and FFR functionality will be a standard feature for all future generations, including the ILUMIEN OPTIS Mobile System and OPTIS Integrated System.

11.2 ILUMIEN OPTIS MOBILE SYSTEM

This section introduces the key components of the ILUMIEN OPTIS Mobile System (Figure 11.2)—the OCT imaging engine and DOC, and the functionality of the mobile console.

TABLE 11.3

Imaging performance comparison of the LightLab/SJM intravascular OCT systems

	ILUMIEN OPTIS	ILUMIEN	C7xr	M3	M2
OCT technology	FD-OCT	FD-OCT	FD-OCT	TD-OCT	TD-OCT
Light source	Swept source	Swept source	Swept source	SLED	SLED
A-Scan rate	>81 kHz	50.4 kHz	50.4 kHz	4.8 kHz	3.2 kHz
Frame rate	180 fps	100 fps	100 fps	20 fps	16 fps
A-Scan range (tissue)	7.0 mm	7.0 mm	7.0 mm	4.6 mm	4.6 mm
Axial resolution (tissue)	≤20 µm	≤20 µm	≤20 µm	≤20 µm	≤20 µm
Maximum pullback range	75 mm	50 mm	50 mm	55 mm	55 mm
Maximum pullback speed	36 mm/s	25 mm/s	25 mm/s	2 mm/s	2 mm/s
Lateral resolution	25–60 µm	25–60 µm	25–60 µm	25–60 µm	25–60 µm
Minimum optical sensitivity	90 dB	90 dB	90 dB	90 dB	90 dB
FFR integration	Yes	Yes	No	No	No

Note: SLED, superluminescent diode.

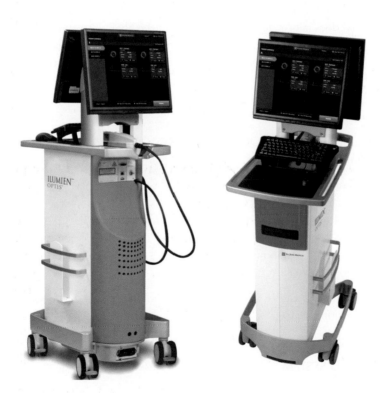

Figure 11.2 ILUMIEN OPTIS Mobile System.

11.2.1 Imaging engine

The OCT imaging engine contains a swept source to produce wavelength-swept near-infrared light in 1.3 μm, a reference arm module to provide the reference optical signal matching the path length and polarization to the optical signal from the sample arm (DOC), an optical module to generate the optical interference signals and clock signals, and a high speed electro-optical (EO) circuit to provide balanced photodetection and clock generation. The backscattered light from the tissue is collected by the imaging catheter, interfered with by the reference light in the optical module, and converted into an electrical signal by the EO circuit as an output of the imaging engine. The electrical signals are then acquired by the data acquisition system (DAS) and the signal and imaging processing is performed by the PC in the system.

11.2.2 Driver-motor and optical controller

The DOC provides bedside control of the most important OCT imaging functions. It is designed to be placed in a sterile bag close to the patient on the catheterization table. Functioning as the sample arm of the OCT imaging system, the DOC provides the interface between the imaging engine and the imaging catheter. Additionally, it provides the high-speed rotation or pullback of the catheter to perform 3D OCT imaging. A fiber-optic rotary joint (FORJ) driven by a high-speed electric motor provides the optical interface between the stationary OCT engine and the rotating imaging catheter. The FORJ-motor assembly is controlled by a stepper motor-based translation stage to perform the pullback. When the operator inserts and locks the outer shell of the catheter into a mating connector on the DOC, the internal optical connection is made automatically. Since the outer shell does not rotate and the pullback of the fiber-optic core of the catheter is performed internally, no moving parts are exposed to the patient or operator during imaging acquisition. The built-in control panel on the DOC provides a simplified interface to execute basic imaging acquisition commands in real time. Table 11.4 lists the functionality of the DOC.

11.2.3 Mobile console

In addition to the imaging engine and DOC, the ILUMIEN OPTIS Mobile System includes the following components integrated into a mobile cart:

- Two monitors (operator side and physician side)
- An isolation transformer
- Aortic pressure and PressureWire receivers (FFR option)
- Wi-Box (FFR option)
- A computer, a keyboard, and a mouse
- A power cable

The detailed functionality of the ILUMIEN OPTIS Mobile System can be found in "ILUMIEN™ OPTIS™ System: Instructions for Use."[1]

11.3 OPTIS INTEGRATED SYSTEM

The OPTIS Integrated System (Figure 11.3) is built into the catheter lab so that OCT and the FFR are immediately available without the need to find, connect, position, and power-on a mobile console. This

TABLE 11.4
DOC controls on ILUMIEN OPTIS Mobile System and OPTIS Integrated System

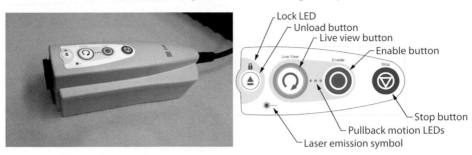

Lock LED	• *Off* when the imaging catheter is not loaded.
	• *Blinking* when loading or unloading the imaging catheter.
	• *On* when the imaging catheter is loaded.
Unload	Press to unload the imaging catheter.
Live View	Press to switch between Standby View and Live View.
Enable	Press to enable recording.
Stop	Press to stop imaging catheter motion and turn off laser output.
Pullback motion LEDs	• *Off* when the imaging catheter is stationary.
	• *Blinks* during pullback.
Laser emission symbol	Illuminated when laser output is on (whenever the system is in Live Scanning mode).

Note: LED, light-emitting diode.

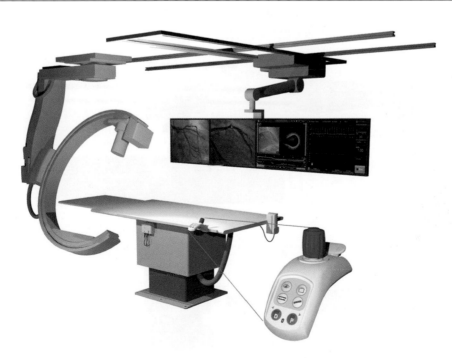

Figure 11.3 OPTIS Integrated System.

section introduces the architectural design of the system, as well as the key components, including the control room cabinet, remoting cable, DOC holster, tableside controller, and mobile workstation, and discusses the installation options.

11.3.1 Architectural design

The OPTIS Integrated System allows the sterile operator to control system functions during image acquisition and review, tightening the linkage between physiological and anatomical assessment with the FFR and OCT and subsequent therapeutic actions. The integrated system offers all the imaging and analysis capabilities of the ILUMIEN OPTIS Mobile System, with an updated user interface designed for easy viewing and operation from the tableside.

The architectural design of the OPTIS Integrated System (Figure 11.4) includes the following new features:

- Control room cabinet: Housing for the engine and PC that is located outside the procedure room.
- DOC holster: Fixture for holding the DOC while not in use. The holster can be mounted on the table rail or the monitor boom, and includes electrical and optical connections to the engine and PC in the control room, as well as wireless receivers for the FFR, tableside controller, and optional third control point monitor, keyboard, and mouse.
- Remoting cable: Cable that runs between the engine in the system cabinet and the DOC holster in the procedure room to carry electrical and optical signals.
- Tableside controller: Joystick with seven buttons to control acquisition and review from the cath table.
- Mobile workstation: Wirelessly connected monitor, keyboard, and mouse on a mobile cart that can be stationed in the procedure room to allow a nonsterile operator to control system functions.
- ACR hardware: Electronics to support capture of cine videos for the ACR software feature.

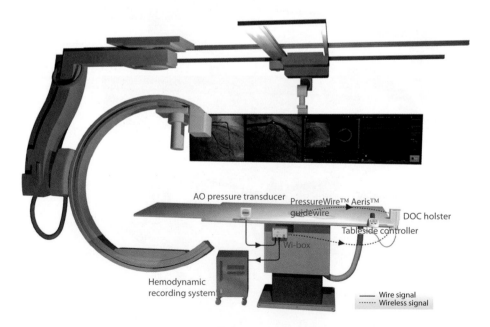

Figure 11.4 OPTIS Integrated System architectural design.

11.3.2 Control room cabinet

The control room cabinet (Figure 11.5) houses the essential components of the system, including the engine, PC, power supply, and USB/video peripheral interface devices. It is intended to be installed in either the control room (under a table) or in the technical closet.

11.3.3 DOC holster

The DOC holster (Figure 11.6) is the central interface in the cath lab. It extends the USB interface from the PC to the DOC, tableside controller, and FFR receivers. The holster is physically connected to the control room cabinet over the 27 m long remoting cable, which carries electrical and optical fiber cables. The holster provides power, as well as optical signals, to the DOC over a 2.7 m cable.

The DOC holster also provides USB power and a control interface to the tableside controller, when the tableside controller is configured in USB mode. It also houses the USB connection to the FFR receivers behind a rear cover with user or installer accessibility.

11.3.4 Remoting cable

The remoting cable is a 27 m long EO hybrid cable that is used to extend the optical signal and power from the control room cabinet to the DOC holster. The cable carries a power cable, along with optical fibers, for the OCT imaging system.

11.3.5 Tableside controller

The tableside controller (Figure 11.7) allows users or physicians to operate the C8i system at the procedural table. The tableside controller integrates a joystick controller for x-y motion and an Enter button, which functions similar to a mouse. It also incorporates a keypad for navigating through the different menu options provided by the application.

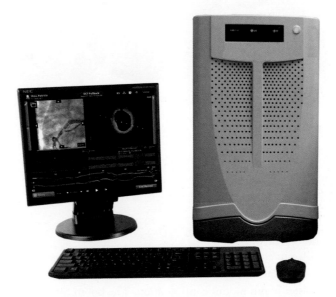

Figure 11.5 OPTIS Integrated System cabinet and control room components.

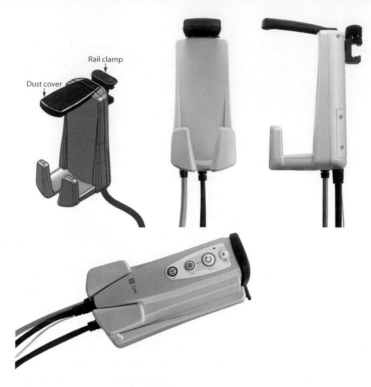

Figure 11.6 DOC holster.

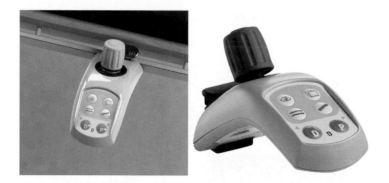

Figure 11.7 Tableside controller.

The tableside controller can connect and communicate to the Holster via USB or Bluetooth mode. During Bluetooth mode, the tableside controller requires a 5 V power supply connecting to its USB input as a source of power.

11.3.6 Installation options (boom vs. table mount)

The DOC holster is typically attached on the patient procedure table rail so the physician can have direct access to the DOC. In some installations, the DOC holster may be installed directly onto the monitor boom, which is called the DOC holster boom mount configuration. The boom mount configuration is intended to make more space on the procedure table rail when OCT is not in use during the procedure.

11.4   OCT APPLICATION SOFTWARE

After the OCT images are acquired, the images are immediately stored as a data set in the system and the user can review the set in the same OCT application software or export the data to other locations. The OCT application software allows the user to review the recorded OCT images with various visualization modes, including B-Mode, L-Mode, and lumen profile displays, as well as 3D visualization of the pullback data sets. This section introduces these different visualization modes and the data storage and export options.

11.4.1   B-Mode, L-Mode, and lumen profile displays

When reviewing the recorded images, the image window shows a cross section of the pullback or the still frame (B-Mode) and an approximate lateral representation of the vessel (L-Mode), as shown in Figure 11.8. By clicking the playback control or moving the current frame indicator (yellow-green bar) in the L-Mode panel, the user can review B-Mode frame by frame to evaluate the depth-resolved structure of the vessel. The image window also allows the user to make measurements, calculations, and text annotations on each B-Mode frame, as well as take a snapshot or export the frames of interest (Table 11.5).

During the OCT pullback recording, the system captures evenly spaced cross section images and uses them to construct a lateral view of the vessel anatomy. The lateral view is shown in the L-Mode display in the lower portion of the screen, and the distal portion of the recording is to the left. The yellow-green bar in the image window is the cut-plane indicator, and the lateral view shown in the L-Mode display can be changed by clicking and dragging this indicator. L-Mode is only available with pullback and stationary recording and not with still images.

Once the OCT images are acquired, the system automatically creates a trace of the lumen contour on each frame. Users can review the lumen profile using the minimum lumen area (MLA) controls, and values for the OCT recording can be displayed on top of the L-Mode view. This feature can provide lesion characteristics and information that helps stent sizing assessment. Table 11.6 shows the lumen profile display with the MLA controls' overview.

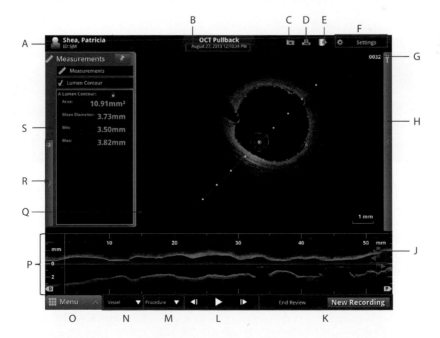

Figure 11.8 Image window with standard B-Mode visualization and the display overview.

TABLE 11.5

OCT Image window functionality

Function	Description
A. Patient name and ID	
B. Recording date and time	
C. Capture button	Save the current frame.
D. Print button	Print the current frame to file.
E. Export button	Click to open the Export Wizard.
F. Setting button	Click to open the Setting menu.
G. Frame number	Only visible on a pause recording.
H. Tool panel	Measurement and Annotation tools.
I. Bookmark control	Add or remove bookmarks to the L-Mode view.
J. End review/new recording	Close the current window and return to Patient Summary menu.
K. Playback control	Control the playback of OCT recording.
L. Procedure list	A drop-down list of procedures to describe this recording.
M. Vessel list	A drop-down list of vessels to describe this recording.
N. Menu	Display the context-sensitive menu.
O. L-Mode view	A lateral representation of the vessel.
P. Image window	A cross-sectional view of the vessel.
Q. View menu	Advanced display and lumen profile submenu.
R. Measurement panel	List of measurements from the current image.

TABLE 11.6

MLA controls

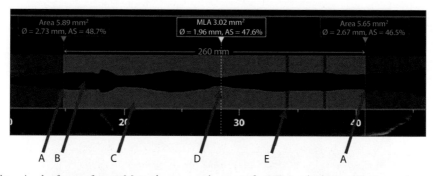

A. *Distal and proximal reference frames*: Move these to set the range for MLA calculation. The system's search for an MLA occurs on frames between the distal and proximal reference frames.

B. The lumen area is colored black.

C. Where the system has high confidence in the contour of the lumen area, or where the contour has been accepted by the user, the section is colored brown.

D. *Calculated MLA*: The dashed line indicates the position of the MLA between the distal and proximal reference frames (A).

E. Where the system has low confidence in the contour of the lumen area, the section is colored red. These frames are not considered in the MLA search.

11.4.2 3D visualization

The high imaging speed of the current systems allows users to acquire pullback images with low motion artifact so that the 3D visualization can provide more structural information on the vessels from different orientations. The OCT application software builds in advanced display modes so the users can review the OCT recordings in 3D Tissue mode and 3D Lumen mode. The 3D Tissue mode renders the cross-sectional OCT frames along the pullback into a 3D volume, which shows the 3D tissue structure of the vessel. Table 11.7 shows an overview of the 3D Tissue mode.

The 3D Lumen mode adds a 3D representation of the lumen contours drawn on each frame, as shown in Figure 11.9. If the MLA is calculated prior to activating the 3D Lumen mode, the distal reference, proximal reference, and MLA frames would also be displayed. These 3D visualization modes can help the user perform qualitative and quantitative evaluation of vascular morphology in the vessels.

TABLE 11.7
3D tissue controls

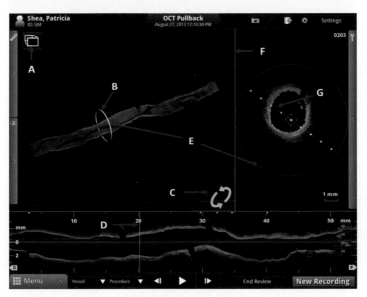

A. *View mode*: Click to toggle between *Window* mode (shown above) and *Full Screen* mode. Also available as a button on the tableside controller.

B. *Current frame indicator* (3D view): Scroll the mouse wheel (or twist the *navigation controller*) to change the cut plane as shown in the L-Mode. This also changes the frame displayed in the cross-sectional view.

C. *Cut-plane rotation hotspot*: Place the cursor over the hotspot and rotate the mouse wheel to change the cut plane as shown in the L-Mode.

D. *Current frame indicator* (L-Mode view): Click and drag to change the frame shown.

E. The 3D view and cross-sectional view relate to each other as follows: The solid lines in the cross-sectional view represent the rendered half of the vessel image in 3D. The dashed lines in the cross-sectional view represent the open, or unrendered, half of the vessel image in 3D. The blue and yellow colors are for location referencing among the views.

F. Click and drag the divider bar side to side to change the size of the 3D display versus the cross section view.

G. *Cut-plane indicator*: The cut plane is shown as a solid line in the cross-sectional view. Click and drag this to change the lateral view shown in the L-Mode display.

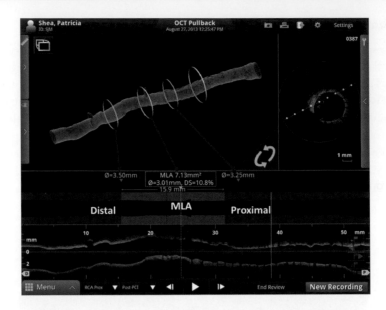

Figure 11.9 MLA frames in 3D lumen display.

11.4.3 Data management

All the OCT recordings are automatically stored as raw OCT files after the image acquisition is completed. The software is able to export, import, and manage the OCT files. Files can be exported in native file format (raw OCT format), a standard graphic file format (standard format), or DICOM format. Exported files can be saved on a CD/DVD or external USB device, or exported to a DICOM storage server. The user can choose whether to delete files after transfer or keep them on the system.

If the native (raw OCT) file format is chosen, every feature of the OCT file will be exported and the files can be imported into another ILUMIEN, ILUMIEN OPTIS Mobile, or OPTIS Integrated System, or an offline review workstation (ORW), where the files can be reviewed and manipulated. An exported OCT file contains exactly the same data as the original file, including any measurements and annotation additions, all patient information associated with each file, and system diagnostic information to help diagnose possible imaging quality problems.

If standard file formats are chosen (AVI, compressed AVI, or multipage TIFF for recordings, and JPEG, TIFF, or BMP for images), the images can be used in computer applications outside the system, but cannot be imported into an ILUMIEN System, an ILUMIEN OPTIS Mobile System, an OPTIS Integrated System, or an ORW.

11.5 ANGIO COREGISTRATION SOFTWARE

ACR is the new feature that allows the user to align the angiography and OCT recording, so OCT frames correlate with the corresponding angiography position. ACR is currently included in the software package of the OPTIS Integrated System. This functionality allows the users to more easily determine their position in the OCT relative to the lesion, and assists in stent location and placement. This section introduces the operating principle; the specifications, including the accuracy and execution time; and the guided workflow of the ACR software.

11.5.1 Operating principle

The OCT/ACR tool is a hardware and software enhancement to the ILUMIEN OPTIS Imaging Systems that allows the user to visualize and manipulate the position of OCT image data on coregistered angiography images. ACR is designed to be compatible with a wide range of installed x-ray systems in the world, and can work with OCT imaging in both Survey mode and High Resolution mode. OCT/ACR software enables visualization of the position of an OCT image on a corresponding angiography image acquired at a similar point in time. To perform ACR, the user must acquire a cine sequence during an OCT pullback. The key for accurate coregistration is the ability to spatially locate the OCT imaging lens throughout the cine sequence.

11.5.2 Guided workflow

The OCT/ACR software provides a comprehensive guided workflow (Figure 11.10) when reviewing OCT recordings with coregistered angiography so that the user can easily perform the coregistration by choosing two or more control points in the angiography images. The OCT/ACR process can be completed with the following steps:

1. Set the first (distal) control point by placing the cursor in the vessel of interest, on or near the RO part of the guidewire, and clicking once (Figure 11.10a). A white control point and Step 2 of the ACR guidance are displayed.
2. Moving distal to proximal, set at least one additional control point by placing the cursor in the vessel of interest, near the guide catheter tip, and clicking once. An additional white control point is

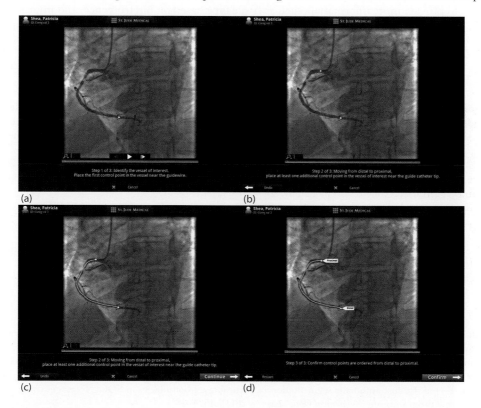

(a)   (b)   (c)   (d)

Figure 11.10 Guided OCT/ACR workflow. (a) First control point set. (b) At least one additional control point near the catheter tip set. (c) Trace line of the vessel of interest connects control points. (d) Coregistration complete.

displayed (Figure 11.10b). The system draws a line that traces the vessel of interest and connects the control points (Figure 11.10c). The Continue button is displayed.

3. Verify that the trace is in the vessel of interest. Click the Continue button. ACR guidance, Step 3, is displayed.

4. Click the Confirm button to accept the path and direction (distal to proximal) within the vessel of interest. The "Please wait for co-registration" screen is displayed, while the system correlates the angiography with the OCT frames. When the coregistration is complete, the "Co-registration completed successfully" screen is displayed (Figure 11.10d).

11.6   CONCLUSION

The ILUMIEN OPTIS Mobile System and OPTIS Integrated System provide the PCI Optimization platforms with intravascular OCT imaging and FFR technology. Incorporated with ACR capability, the OPTIS Integrated System allows the user to visualize the position of OCT image data on angiography images, tightening the linkage between anatomical assessment with OCT and subsequent therapeutic actions.

With the advance of OCT technologies, the OCT imaging speed can be increased so that the total acquisition time can be shortened, resulting in the reduction of contrast usage during OCT imaging and reduced motion artifact from heartbeat. Polarization diversity detection techniques[24] can also be implemented into the OCT system to provide more information, such as tissue type based on birefringence, and improve the image quality. These technologies are expected to further extend the clinical utility of OCT for PCI optimization.

REFERENCES

1. St. Jude Medical. ILUMIEN™ OPTIS™ System: Instructions for use. Rev. A. St. Paul, MN: St. Jude Medical.
2. St. Jude Medical. OPTIS™ Integrated System: Instructions for use. Rev. A. St. Paul, MN: St. Jude Medical.
3. Takada K et al. New measurement system for fault location in optical waveguide devices based on an interferometric technique. *Applied Optics* 1987;26:1603–8.
4. Youngquist R et al. Optical coherence-domain reflectometry. *Optics Letters* 1987;12:158–60.
5. Gilgen HH et al. Submillimeter optical reflectometry. *IEEE Journal of Lightwave Technology* 1989;7:1225–33.
6. Huang D et al. Optical coherence tomography. *Science* 1991;254:1778–81.
7. Swanson EA et al. High-speed optical coherence domain reflectometry. *Optics Letters* 1992;17:151–3.
8. Choma MA et al. Sensitivity advantage of swept source and Fourier domain optical coherence tomography. *Optics Express* 2003;11:2183–9.
9. de Boer JF et al. Improved signal-to-noise ratio in spectral-domain compared with time-domain optical coherence tomography. *Optics Letters* 203;28:2067–9.
10. Leitgeb R et al. Performance of Fourier domain vs. time domain optical coherence tomography. *Optics Express* 2003;11:889–94.
11. Cense B et al. Ultrahigh-resolution high-speed retinal imaging using spectral-domain optical coherence tomography. *Optics Express* 2004;12:2435–47.
12. Wojtkowski M et al. Three-dimensional retinal imaging with high-speed ultrahigh-resolution optical coherence tomography. *Ophthalmology* 2005;112:1734–46.
13. Potsaid B et al. Ultrahigh speed spectral/Fourier domain OCT ophthalmic imaging at 70,000 to 312,500 axial scans per second. *Optics Express* 2008;16:15149–69.
14. LaRocca F et al. Robust automatic segmentation of corneal layer boundaries in SDOCT images using graph theory and dynamic programming. *Biomedical Optics Express* 2011;2:1524–38.
15. Chinn SR et al. Optical coherence tomography using a frequency-tunable optical source. *Optics Letters* 1997;22:340–2.
16. Yun SH et al. High-speed optical frequency-domain imaging. *Optics Express* 2003;11:2953–63.

17. Huber R et al. Unidirectional swept laser sources for optical coherence tomography at 370,000 lines/s. *Optics Letters* 2006;31:2975–7.
18. Adler DC et al. Phase-sensitive optical coherence tomography at up to 370,000 lines per second using buffered Fourier domain mode-locked lasers. *Optics Letters* 2007;32:626–8.
19. Tsai T-H et al. Ultrahigh speed endoscopic optical coherence tomography using micromotor imaging catheter and VCSEL technology. *Biomedical Optics Express* 2013;4:1119–32.
20. Brezinski ME et al. Optical coherence tomography for optical biopsy. Properties and demonstration of vascular pathology. *Circulation* 1996;93:1206–13.
21. St. Jude Medical. C7 Dragonfly™ imaging catheter: Instructions for use. Rev. E. St. Paul, MN: St. Jude Medical.
22. St. Jude Medical. Dragonfly™ JP/Duo imaging catheter: Instructions for use. Rev. C. St. Paul, MN: St. Jude Medical.
23. St. Jude Medical. Dragonfly™ OPTIS™ imaging catheter: Instructions for use. Rev. A. St. Paul, MN: St. Jude Medical.
24. Wang Z et al. Depth-encoded all-fiber swept source polarization sensitive OCT. *Biomedical Optics Express* 2014;5:2931–49.

Chapter 12

Terumo OFDI system

Kenji Kaneko, Tetsuya Fusazaki, and Takayuki Okamura

12.1 INTRODUCTION

Terumo's intravascular optical frequency-domain imaging (OFDI) system aims to acquire cross-sectional images of the coronary artery lumen and the surface of the vessel wall. Terumo's OFDI system is a composite of an imaging catheter, FastView, and imaging console, LUNAWAVE (Figure 12.1a–c). FastView is connected to a motor drive unit (MDU) of LUNAWAVE when it is in use. Infrared light generated in LUNAWAVE is delivered to the tip of FastView via an optical fiber embedded in a rotational torque wire (driveshaft). Light is emitted through a miniature ball lens (Figure 12.2) located at the distal end of the driveshaft, which emits light to the target observation point of the vessel wall. Backscattered light from tissue and/or the implanted device is collected and transferred back to LUNAWAVE to construct an OFDI image and display it on the monitor. The MDU rotates the driveshaft to allow the system to acquire cross-sectional intravascular imaging.

12.2 FASTVIEW IMAGING CATHETER

12.2.1 Components and architecture

Two major components are the driveshaft and catheter sheath. The driveshaft rotates within a catheter sheath to acquire a round vessel image. Automated mechanical pullback by the MDU lets the system acquire a longitudinal vessel image.

12.2.2 Clinical setup and compatibility

FastView is a 0.0014-in. compatible rapid exchange-type imaging catheter, of which the short monorail lumen length is 20 mm. The usable length of FastView is 137 cm, and the profile of the imaging window is 2.6 and 3.2 Fr for its proximal spiral shaft. A 100 cm supreme-quality hydrophilic coating from its tip realizes excellent crossability and trackability in the coronary artery. The inner diameter of the compatible guiding catheter is ≥1.78 mm (0.070 in.) (Figure 12.3a and b).

Two radiopaque markers are a key enhancement of its usability under fluoroscopic guidance to let physicians know where the tip of the catheter is and where the OFDI image acquisition is taking place. The tip

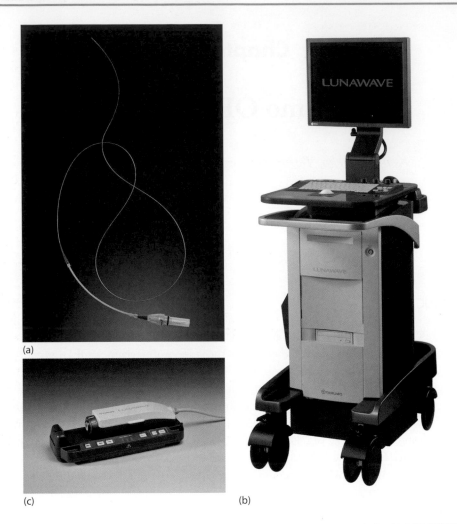

(a)

(c)

(b)

Figure 12.1 (a) FastView OFDI imaging catheter. (b) LUNAWAVE OFDI imaging console. (c) LUNAWAVE MDU.

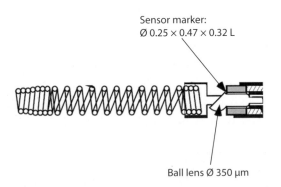

Figure 12.2 Schema of FastView ball lens.

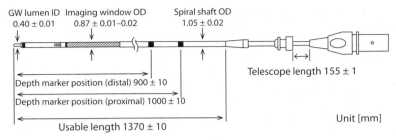

GW lumen ID   Imaging window OD   Spiral shaft OD
0.40 ± 0.01   0.87 ± 0.01–0.02   1.05 ± 0.02

Telescope length 155 ± 1

Depth marker position (distal) 900 ± 10

Depth marker position (proximal) 1000 ± 10

Usable length 1370 ± 10

Unit [mm]

Hydrophilic coating length from tip to 1000 ± 100 mm

(a)

Distal radiopaque marker

1 mm

5 mm

Length of guidewire insertion tube: 20 mm

(b)

Figure 12.3 (a) Dimensions of FastView catheter. (b) Close-up of the distal tip of the catheter and the closed inner lumen architecture. GW, guidewire; ID, inner diameter; OD, outer diameter.

marker is placed 5 mm from its distal tip end, and the lens marker (second marker) is placed at the site where light is emitted.

FastView is compatible only with LUNAWAVE. FastView is packaged with a sterile bag (MDU cover) that covers up the nonsterile MDU to allow it to be placed on a sterile field.

12.2.3 Characteristics of FastView

The following five points are the main characteristics of FastView:

1. *Plug-and-play and noiseless design for less stress imaging.* Unlike other intravascular ultrasound (IVUS) and optical coherence tomography (OCT) catheters, FastView does not need to purge its inner lumen by saline or contrast media, because reflection from the sheath surface is highly restricted by its design and coating technology. This priming-free design lets physicians connect easily, and does not allow reverse flow of blood to its inner lumen, which would cause degradation of the image quality and/or an air bubble artifact.
2. *Excellent trackability catheter and short tip design to image more distally.* The catheter profile is very small and flexible, and the well-known Terumo's hydrophilic coating realizes excellent trackability to distal sites. The short lens–tip distance, only 24 mm, helps physicians to acquire images from further points of the vessel.
3. *High-performance torque wire leads to stable and "circular" image.* With well-developed coiling technology and architecture, the driveshaft achieves high torque deliverability from the MDU to the distal lens tip. The driveshaft realizes very few nonuniform rotational distortions (NURDs), even with high-speed rotations of 158 frames/s.

4. *Lens marker, principle of the angio coregistration system.* A radiopaque marker is made of an alloy of platinum and iridium, which is well observed under fluoroscopy. The lens marker is placed at the miniature ball lens. This design lets physicians know where imaging will start in the angiography, and the acquired OFDI image can be traced on angiography by using the angio coregistration function to have an easier understanding of the vessel anatomy and tissue character.

5. *Whole-vessel scanning.* The driveshaft is telescopically pulled back by the MDU, which has a maximum length of 150 mm. This is the longest pullback length in current commercially available intravascular imaging systems. For instance, its maximum length can cover from distal to proximal of the long right coronary artery (RCA).

12.3 LUNAWAVE OFDI IMAGING CONSOLE

LUNAWAVE, Terumo's OFDI imaging console, has been commercially available since April 2012 in Europe and since April 2013 in Japan. Besides Europe and Japan, it has been launched in Southeast Asia, Oceania, the Middle East, North Africa, and South America. The characteristics of LUNAWAVE are its high-resolution cross-sectional imaging, high signal-to-noise ratio (S/N), and high-speed long pullback with a dedicated imaging catheter, FastView. Its software is utilized to support percutaneous coronary intervention (PCI) procedures. In this section, the product characteristics and utility of PCI are covered.

12.3.1 LUNAWAVE imaging technologies

12.3.1.1 Polygon scanner wavelength filter

A wavelength swept-source laser is the key component of Fourier-domain OCT and OFDI. There are a variety of swept-source laser technologies, such as the microelectromechanical systems, Fourier domain mode locking laser, and vertical cavity surface emitting laser. Aiming to acquire a high S/N and stable OFDI image, a Polygon scanner wavelength filter is selected for the LUNAWAVE light source, characterizing low noise and a constant- or stable-output swept-source laser.

12.3.1.2 Sensitivity peak shift

OFDI delivers infrared light to the coronary artery through a thin optical fiber enclosed in an imaging catheter and emits to the vessel wall from its distal tip. Backscattered light from tissue is collected by the imaging catheter. Collected light is delivered back to the system and amplified by the interference principle. Generally, backscattered light from tissue is about $1/10^{10}$ of the input light intensity, and signal from the deep part is even more attenuated as light travels in the tissue, resulting in an image of less penetration depth.

OFDI improved this issue by shifting the sensitivity peak from the origin of the image (center of the image) to about 2.5 mm in depth, using a featured module inside the imaging console. Sensitivity peak shifting allowed for high S/N distribution in its imaging range and realized deeper penetration depth imaging.

12.3.1.3 Laser safety mechanisms

LUNAWAVE has double safety mechanisms that are designed to ensure the catheter does not emit a laser when it is not scanning. This design allows LUNAWAVE to be categorized in the safest category, Class 1 of the laser safety standard IEC 60825-1, although it realizes high-intensity laser emission to achieve a high-S/N image while scanning.

12.3.2 Reliability

12.3.2.1 Data protection and backup system

LUNAWAVE carries two data storages mirroring one another. Even if one storage malfunctions, LUNAWAVE can salvage data from the other.

12.3.3 Image acquisition setups

12.3.3.1 Pullback condition setting

Depending on a patient's condition and the lesion length, the blood removal time (flush duration) and image acquisition length change. To adapt to each situation, the pullback speed setting is selectable from 0, 5, 10, 15, 20, 25, 30, or 40 mm/s and the pullback length can be set to up to 150 mm preliminarily or can be terminated manually. Precise adjustments of pullback conditions help to reduce the total amount of contrast media as the flushing agent. To avoid confusion during a procedure, LUNAWAVE has three preset shortcuts that allow one to select frequently used conditions. Shortcuts would be applied to function keys (F1, F2, and F3) on console keyboard and make the procedure simpler.

12.3.3.2 Pullback speed and frame pitch

Since the frame rate of LUNAWAVE is constant at 158 frames/s, the frame pitch changes as the pullback speed changes. The frame pitch dependency versus the pullback speed of LUNAWAVE is shown in Table 12.1. In the case of three-dimensional (3D) reconstruction, the frame pitch should be as small as possible to achieve a higher-resolution image. On the other hand, a slower pullback speed leads to more motion artifacts caused by the heartbeat. This trade-off should be considered before acquiring OFDI pullback.[1]

12.3.3.3 Automatic injector setup: flush rate and volume

The image acquisition time depends on the length and speed of the pullback, although generally the acquisition time is around 2–3 seconds. Since infrared light is highly attenuated within blood, OFDI requires removal of blood while images are acquired. A flushing agent such as contrast media is injected around 3–4 seconds in general. Although the required injection rate depends on the geography of the vessels, the most effective factors are the position and coaxiality of the guiding catheter while injecting. When the guiding catheter tip is faced as parallel as possible to the longitude of the vessel, blood will be removed in an even smaller amount of

TABLE 12.1
Frame pitch dependency on pullback speed

Pullback speed (mm/s)	Frame pitch (mm)
0	–
5	0.032
10	0.063
15	0.095
20	0.127
25	0.158
30	0.190
40	0.253

flushing agent. To confirm the position and coaxiality, test flush with a small amount of flush media (around 2 cc). In most cases, 3.0 cc/s for the RCA and 3.5 cc/s for the left coronary artery (LCA) are adequate rates of injection, although adjustment of the injection conditions should be considered case by case.

12.3.4 Stent implantation supporting software

12.3.4.1 Preinterventional diagnosis

Selection of the landing zone of the drug-eluting stent may be optimized by OFDI observation. Not only measurement of the lesion length and lumen size, but also tissue characterization of the plaque is well determined, especially in the identification of fibrous, fibroatheroma, and fibrocalcific plaque. Frequently observed characteristics in vulnerable plaque, such as plaque rupture, erosion, thrombus, thin-cap fibroatheroma, and microvessel, are visualized by OFDI and allow physicians to determine an interventional strategy from the acquired OFDI images to select the stent size and length and place to deploy.

The LUNAWAVE measurement function is designed to support stent sizing and landing zone selection (Video 12.1).

12.3.4.2 Area measurement

The lumen, media, and any other cross-sectional region are measureable by area measurement functions. Lumen and stent measurement may be automatically traced by one click. Traced contours may be adjusted manually. The centroid of the traced line, area, maximum and minimum diameter, and mean diameter will be automatically calculated and shown on the display.

12.3.4.3 Length measurement

The length between any two frames is measured. While measuring length, cross-sectional images of two dedicated frames are also displayed, the so-called X-View mode, to observe both the distal and proximal reference sites simultaneously (Video 12.2). This measurement function can also be utilized for landing zone selection. For example, in considering to deploy a 24 mm stent, prepare a 24 mm length measurement result, select the result bar, and move along the longitudinal view to observe the landing frames of the stent (Video 12.3).

These measurement results will be saved automatically; no extra attention is required to archive results with this system.

12.3.4.4 Angio coregistration

Since the stenting procedure is held under fluoroscopic observation, coregistration of the OFDI image to angiography is important. In order to trace the location of the cross-sectional OFDI image in angiography, the angio coregistration function is equipped with LUNAWAVE.

Angio coregistration works only when an angio image is input to the system via a dedicated port. Angio images are archived during OFDI pullback. Automatically archived angio images are displayed on the monitor when the Angio button is selected. A radiopaque lens marker is located at the edge of the miniature ball lens of FastView; spatial error between the ball lens and marker is negligible. The location of the cross-sectional image is identifiable by tracing the lens marker on the angio coregistration window (Figure 12.4).

If angio coregistration is active, two angio coregistered images are displayed during the length measurement with cross-sectional images. Since the display is divided by four (two cross-sectional images and two angio coregistration images), the visibility of each angio image is degraded. By double-clicking the image, these divided sections can be enlarged and help observation of the lens marker (Figure 12.5 and Video 12.4).

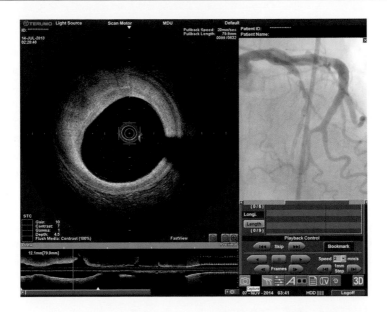

Figure 12.4 Angio coregistration user interface.

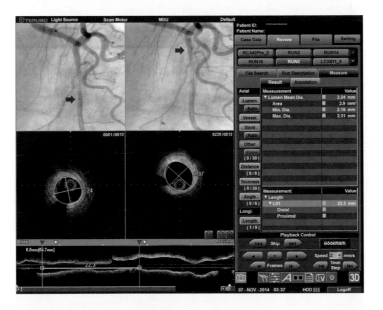

Figure 12.5 Lumen and length measurement in X-View mode for stent planning. Red arrows: lens marker of the FastView catheter.

12.3.5 PCI procedure evaluation

A high-resolution OFDI image clearly visualizes stent malapposition, edge dissection, and protrusion of tissue after implantation. The distance and thickness measurement function allows one to evaluate stent apposition by a simple operation, and the dual-review mode (coregistration of two OFDI pullbacks) helps one to understand the procedural effect on the site.

12.3.5.1 Distance and thickness measurement

These functions measure the distance between two points and help us to evaluate the fibrous cap thickness of plaque, postprocedure stent malapposition, and neointimal thickness in follow-up. Distance is measurement of selected two points on a cross-sectional image. The thickness measurement requires a preliminary lumen measurement, and by selecting a dedicated point on an image, the distance from the point to the lumen contour can be measured automatically. This line is along the centroid of the lumen measurement. The thickness measurement is useful if one is measuring the distance of multiple points to the lumen contour, especially stent strut apposition and neointimal coverage evaluation since continuous measurement is supported in this function (Figure 12.6). All these measurement results can be exported to a spreadsheet (CSV file format).

12.3.5.2 Dual-review mode

LUNAWAVE supports the comparison of any two different pullbacks at the same time with a dual-review mode. This function allows one to play back two pullbacks individually and while synchronizing. Comparison between two pullbacks to confirm the procedure and baseline follow-ups is effective for this function (Figure 12.7).

12.3.6 Evaluation of bifurcation lesion: 3D OFDI

3D reconstruction supports visualization of the implanted stent strut, especially at the bifurcation lesion (Video 12.4).

12.3.6.1 3D reconstruction

Two main characteristics of the LUNAWAVE 3D function are (1) the stent and guidewire emphasis and the (2) free rotation of the 3D image. The deployed stent and guidewire location are observed online. Since 3D reconstruction uses all intensity data of the cross-sectional image, loss of acquired information is minimized.

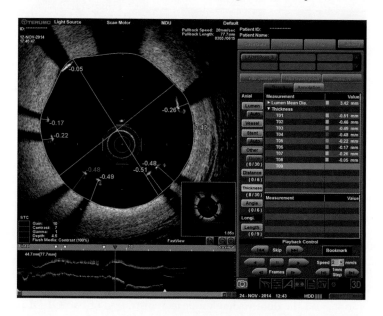

Figure 12.6 Thickness measurement function by continuous clicks to measure the distance from points to the lumen contour.

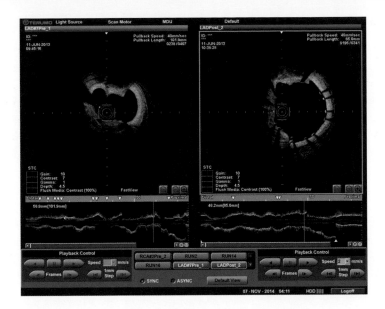

Figure 12.7 Dual-review mode. Example of comparison between pre- and poststenting.

1. The stent highlight function works to detect characteristics of signals from metallic materials. Automatically detected stents and guidewires will be emphasized in the 3D image in a different color (white) to help observation (Figure 12.8a–c). The visualized intensity range in the 3D image is adjustable with two parameters, the window level and window width. By adjusting these parameters, low-intensity noise, such as remaining blood, may be reduced or a detected stent may be selectively visualized (Figure 12.9).

2. The angle between the main vessel and the bifurcation varies from case to case. The degree of freedom in rotation is a preferred characteristic of 3D OFDI. Rotation also helps one to recognize the depth and position relationship of the 3D image.

LUNAWAVE has two different views of 3D images. One is the cutaway view, the so-called vessel view, and the other is the opened vessel view, the carpet view. The carpet view allows one to observe all luminal

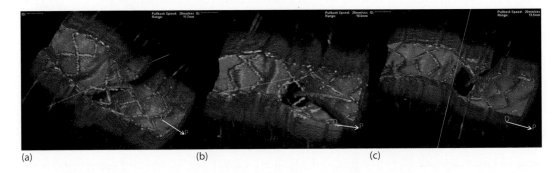

(a) (b) (c)

Figure 12.8 Vessel view examples of (a) unoptimized wire recross, (b) optimized wire recross, and (c) post-KBT in example (b).

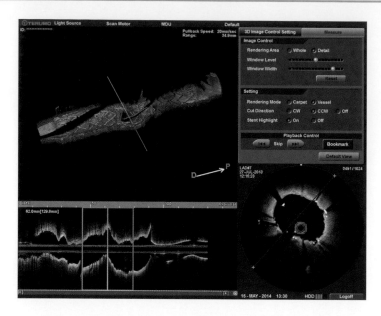

Figure 12.9 Vessel view user interface. The cut plane of 3D image is set by selecting the region of interest in axial image (red line) and longitudinal window (orange and green lines).

information in a simple operation. Since the location of the link near the bifurcation will affect the postballooning stent deformation, an overview observation helps one to foresee the procedure results (Figure 12.10a–c).

12.3.7 File export

LUNAWAVE has various output options in still images and playback movies.

Still images can be a whole-display screenshot, an axial image only, or axial + longitudinal images in BMP or JPEG format.

3D images are also capable being output as still images.

Playback movies can be an axial image only (Video 12.5), axial + longitudinal images (Video 12.6), axial + longitudinal images + angio coregistration (Video 12.7), a dual-review axial image only, or dual-review axial + longitudinal (Video 12.8) images in AVI format.

The DICOM format is also supported in LUNAWAVE. DICOM files can be transferred to a picture archiving and communication system server and external media as USB storage and CD/DVD media. DICOM modalities supported by LUNAWAVE are ultrasound (US), IVUS, OCT, and intravascular optical coherence tomography.

12.4 CASE REPORT: USEFULNESS OF OFDI-GUIDED PCI FOR THE SEPARATED PROXIMAL AND MID–LEFT ANTERIOR DESCENDING ARTERY LESIONS

Tetsuya Fusazaki

A 54-year-old male, admitted for chest pain and who was on effort angina, revealed severe stenosis on coronary angiography (CAG) at the proximal and mid–left anterior descending artery (LAD). PCI was performed by a left transradial approach using a 6 Fr guiding catheter. Target lesions were separated into the

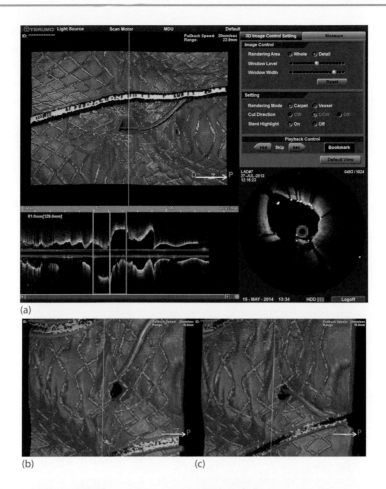

Figure 12.10 (a) Carpet view user interface. Carpet view examples of (b) unoptimized wire recross and (c) optimized wire recross.

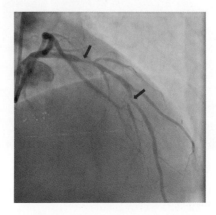

Figure 12.11 Coronary artery angiogram showing severe stenosis at the proximal and mid-LAD (arrows).

proximal and mid-LAD (Figure 12.11). OFDI was performed at the beginning of the procedure in order to obtain precise information to develop a strategy. An OFDI setting of 40 mm/s pullback speed was selected to obtain an image of two lesions with one pullback. This high-speed pullback and the 150 mm maximum pull-back length of the OFDI catheter enable us to obtain a long lesion image with one pullback. This advantage possibly reduces the amount of contrast agent. In the present case, the contrast injection setting was 4.0 cc/s and 10 cc of its amount (Video 12.9).

One of the useful features in the clinical setting of OFDI is the angio coregistration function. The location of the radiopaque marker of the optical sensor displayed in the angiogram can be synchronized with the OFDI longitudinal and cross-sectional view. Measurements of the diameter, area, and lengths of the proximal and distal sites of the lesion on the OFDI can be made by confirming the location of the optical sensor visualized in the angiogram, which could guide the precise positioning of stent implantation. Moreover, the operator can select the stent size easily by using X-View, showing OFDI cross-sectional images and angio images of the proximal and distal positions simultaneously.

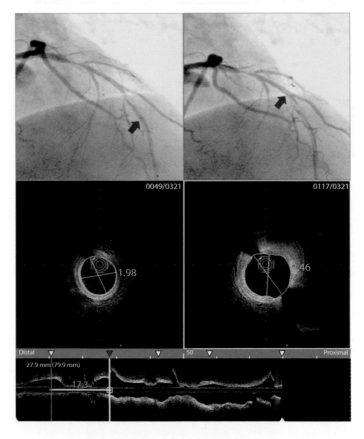

Figure 12.12 Measurement of the mid-LAD lesion by OFDI. The length and diameter of the lesion were measured semi-automatically in a single view. The measurement showed a 2.46 mm lumen diameter at the proximal site of the lesion and a 17.3 mm lesion length. Red arrows: lens marker of the FastView catheter.

The mid-LAD lesion was evaluated as 17 mm in length and 2.5 mm in diameter by OFDI measurement. The optimal proximal landing point was considered to be just distal to the second diagonal branch (Figure 12.12), and a 2.5/18 mm stent was selected. Similarly, the length and diameter of the proximal lesion were measured by OFDI and resulted in a 14 mm lesion length and 3.0 mm diameter of the proximal site of the lesion. The appropriate distal landing point was considered to be just proximal to the first major septal branch (Figure 12.13). Based on these measurement results, a 3.0/18 mm stent was selected in the proximal site by jailing the first diagonal branch. As incomplete strut apposition was confirmed by poststenting OFDI, postdilatation was performed by a noncompliant balloon. The final OFDI visualized the stent apposition well at both sites (Figures 12.14 and 12.15a and b and Video 12.10).

The dual-review mode, which is another unique feature of OFDI, can show two different OFDI cross-sectional images, such as the pre- and post-PCI (Video 12.11). In the present case, stent implantations for two separated lesions at LAD could be performed guided by only one OFDI pullback and the angio coregistration function, which enabled us to use less contrast media.

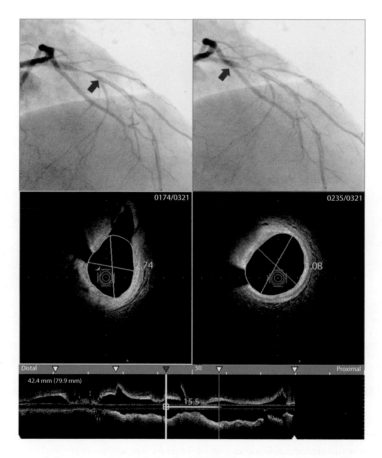

Figure 12.13 Measurement of the proximal LAD lesion by OFDI. The measurement showed a 3.08 mm lumen diameter at the proximal site of the lesion and a 15.5 mm lesion length. Red arrows: lens marker of the FastView catheter.

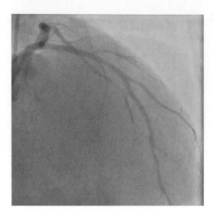

Figure 12.14 Final coronary artery angiogram.

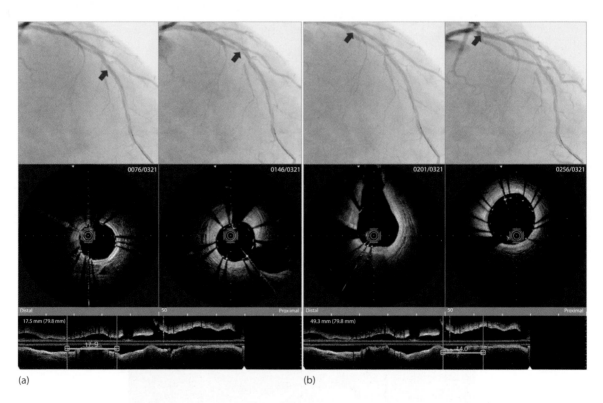

(a)   (b)

Figure 12.15 (a) Final OFDI view of the distal lesion. OFDI revealed the strut apposition well. (b) Final OFDI view of the proximal lesion. OFDI revealed the strut apposition well. Red arrows: lens marker of the FastView catheter.

OFDI-guided PCI is very efficient and convenient because of its various functions, such as long pullback mode, angio coregistration, auto lumen measurement, and length measurement with one window, "X-View mode."

Additionally, the 3D reconstruction function is useful for confirming the struts jailing at the side branch (SB).

12.5 CASE REPORT: USEFULNESS OF 3D OFDI FOR BIFURCATION PCI

Takayuki Okamura

12.5.1 Introduction

3D reconstruction of OCT images with stent strut detection is considered useful for bifurcation PCI.[2,3] We have reported that both the strut configuration in front of the SB orifice and the rewiring position before kissing balloon dilatation (KBD) influenced the incidence of incomplete apposition (ISA) after KBD.[4] Although distal rewiring is generally recommended,[5] choosing the appropriate cell under comprehension of the strut configuration in front of the SB orifice is important. However, it is difficult to recognize the strut configuration in front of the SB orifice with only cross-sectional OCT images. Terumo OFDI equipped the 3D

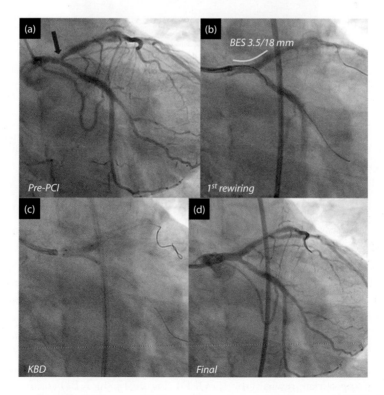

Figure 12.16 Coronary angiography. (a) Prestent. (b) First rewiring after stent deployment. (c) KBD. (d) Final.

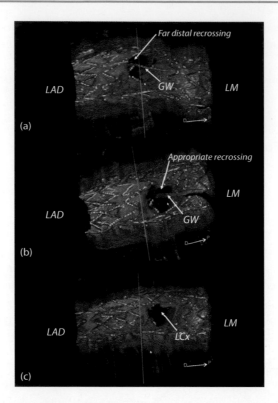

Figure 12.17 3D OFDI. (a) First rewiring. The guidewire (GW) is passed through the far distal cell. (b) Second rewiring. The GW located the appropriate cell for KBD. (c) After KBD. The ostium of the LCx was widely opened and there were no residual struts in front of the LCx ostium. LM, left main trunk.

reconstruction with stent detection. Since 3D OFDI images are reconstructed within 60 seconds, an assessment of the rewiring position is feasible during PCI.

12.5.2 Case

A 69-year-old male, who was on dialysis with effort angina, underwent PCI. CAG revealed a 75% calcified stenosis just proximal to the LAD (Figure 12.16a). The fractional flow reserve (FFR) was 0.76. A 7 Fr backup left 3.5 guiding catheter (Heartrail II) was inserted via the right femoral artery and guidewires were advanced to the LAD and left circumflex artery (LCx). As the pre-OFDI image demonstrated, the calcium was just proximal to the LAD, and rotational atherectomy with a 2.0 mm burr was used. After predilatation with a 3.5 mm noncompliant balloon at 18 atm, a 3.5–18 mm Nobori™ biolimus A9 eluting stent was deployed across the LCx (Figure 12.16b). A second wire was passed to the LCx through the jailing strut. 3D OFDI clearly demonstrated that the second wire passed through the far distal small cell (Figure 12.7a). It was considered a stent deformation after KBD. Second rewiring was attempted to recross more proximally. After confirmation of appropriate rewiring by 3D OFDI (Figure 12.7b), KBD commenced (Figure 12.16c). The final CAG and 3D OFDI revealed an acceptable SB opening without the residual struts at the SB orifice (Figures 12.16d and 12.17c).

12.5.3 Discussion

While the role of KBD was the acquisition of the SB ostial diameter and removal of the stent strut from the SB orifice, KBD could potentially cause the stent deformation, elliptical dilatation of the proximal main vessel, SB injury, etc.[6] In order to achieve optimal KBD, choosing the appropriate cell for rewiring before KBD is important. 3D OFDI might be useful to understand the strut configuration and confirm the rewiring position during PCI. This technology is expected to improve the outcome after bifurcation PCI.

VIDEOS

Video 12.1 Basic stent planning in LUNAWAVE. Decide on the reference site, start measuring the length, and find another reference site. Once proximal and distal references are selected, click the Auto button under the Lumen button. Measurement of the length and lumen size and reference site selection can be smoothly done in a few steps. https://youtu.be/FphDuc2OEbM.

Video 12.2 X-View. Simultaneous observation of OFDI and angio images of reference sites allows smooth stent planning. https://youtu.be/39LyBwdYIdA.

Video 12.3 X-View. Stent landing zone selection may be performed by manipulating the designated length bar to observe both stent edge tissue characters. https://youtu.be/kXtL3lnIqec.

Video 12.4 X-view. Angio window enlargement to improve visibility of the lens marker in a case in which it was to find. https://youtu.be/RdjA2SC0DRw.

Video 12.5 3D reconstruction in both the vessel view and carpet view. https://youtu.be/fVpyESVI25I.

Video 12.6 Example of an axial image of an OFDI playback movie. In this case, residual thrombus after thrombectomy is observed. https://youtu.be/cq_arRLV5hQ.

Video 12.7 Example of an axial + longitudinal image of an OFDI playback movie. In this case, the lesion seems to be diffusely calcified and calcified node-looking character is seen at the proximal vessel. https://youtu.be/DvBSrGKoYLQ.

Video 12.8 Example of an axial + longitudinal image of an OFDI + angio image playback movie. The lens marker in the angio image traces the location of OFDI images. https://youtu.be/HxVmdUhBf_Q.

Video 12.9 Pre-OFDI image. https://youtu.be/6K1bImaPHq0.

Video 12.10 Post-OFDI image. https://youtu.be/aycWHOu8Ka0.

Video 12.11 Dual-review mode of OFDI image. Pre- and post-PCI images can be compared in the same window. https://youtu.be/iUgThNDUnOI.

ACKNOWLEDGMENT

Kenji Kaneko appreciates Professor Shiro Uemura from the Kawasaki Medical School for providing OFDI cases for rewiring, on behalf of the Terumo OFDI group.

DISCLOSURES

FastView and LUNAWAVE are not cleared or approved by the U.S. Food and Drug Administration for use or sale in the United States.

REFERENCES

1. Okamura T et al. High-speed intracoronary optical frequency domain imaging: Implications for three-dimensional reconstruction and quantitative analysis. *EuroIntervention* 2012;7:1216–26.
2. Okamura T et al. Three-dimensional optical coherence tomography assessment of coronary wire re-crossing position during bifurcation stenting. *EuroIntervention* 2011;7:886–7.
3. Farooq V et al. Three-dimensional optical frequency domain imaging in conventional percutaneous coronary intervention: The potential for clinical application. *European Heart Journal* 2013;34:875–85.
4. Okamura T et al. 3D optical coherence tomography: New insights into the process of optimal rewiring of side branches during bifurcational stenting. *EuroIntervention* 2014;10:907–15.
5. Alegría-Barrero E et al. Optical coherence tomography for guidance of distal cell recrossing in bifurcation stenting: Choosing the right cell matters. *EuroIntervention* 2012;8:205–13.
6. Sgueglia GA, Chevalier B. Kissing balloon inflation in percutaneous coronary interventions. *JACC Cardiovascular Interventions* 2012;5:803–11.

Chapter 13

OCT imaging acquisition

Manabu Kashiwagi, Takashi Kubo, Hironori Kitabata, and Takashi Akasaka

13.1 INTRODUCTION

Intracoronary optical coherence tomography (OCT) is a catheter-based imaging technology that employs near-infrared light.[1–4] OCT can provide approximately 10–20 μm axial and 20–40 μm transverse resolutions *in vivo*. These detailed assessments enable us to detect the thin-capped fibroatheromas (TCFAs),[5,6] known as vulnerable plaques,[7] and to evaluate stent failure (e.g., apposition) immediately after coronary stenting and strut coverage at late follow-up.[8–10] OCT has recently contributed to the evaluation of bioresorbable vascular scaffolds (BVSs), which are expected to be the next challenging therapeutic approach for coronary artery disease.[11–13] To date, there are two types of OCT for coronary artery imaging. The first generation is called time-domain (TD) OCT, and the second-generation is called frequency-domain (FD) OCT, also known as optical frequency-domain imaging (OFDI), which has several advantages in interventional cardiology.[14,15] OFDI is designed as a catheter type, like intravascular ultrasound (IVUS). Therefore, it is easier and more conventional compared with the first-generation OCT system. It is expected that detailed information from OFDI will allow us to make better decisions in coronary intervention.[16,17] However, to obtain clear views, there are some matters that require careful attention. Unclear imaging has the potential to lead us to misunderstand the coronary lesions, and subsequently make wrong decisions, resulting in nonoptimized therapies. In this chapter, we focus on how to obtain clearer and more correct OFDI images *in vivo*.

13.2 SYSTEM OF OCT

OCT applies near-infrared light and constructs the images by the interference pattern of reflected light from samples and the reference. Because near-infrared light is attenuated by blood, the target lesion must be cleared from the blood for OCT imaging. We have two types of OCT systems for coronary artery imaging: TD-OCT and OFDI. TD-OCT is a first-generation OCT system, and its commercialized device is developed as a wire-type system. For TD-OCT imaging, there are two methods, the proximal balloon occlusion technique and the nonocclusive technique, to clear blood from the coronary artery.[18,19] In the proximal balloon occlusion technique, an occlusive balloon is placed proximal to the target lesion and then inflated, and the flushing media is injected from the distal tip of the occlusive balloon to clear the site of interest from blood. Compared with FD-OCT (frame rate 150–180 frames/s), the TD-OCT system (frame rate 15–20 frames/s) requires a longer imaging time due to its slow speed of imaging acquisition (pullback speed 2.0–3.0 mm/s) and more complex procedure. Thus, these disadvantages could cause some complications, including heart ischemia, critical arrhythmia, and coronary intima injury by occlusion balloon. The second-generation OCT system, OFDI, has resolved these kinds of problems. The current OFDI can provide a higher frame rate (exceeding 150 frames/s), which is about 10 times that of the TD-OCT system, and enables us to examine the whole coronary artery during one pullback. OFDI systems are commercialized from two manufacturers (St. Jude Medical and Terumo), and both catheters compromise the monorail component. Regarding the clearance of blood from the coronary artery, the continuous coronary flushing technique with contrast media is mainly applied for FD-OCT imaging. Major complications that are reported are ischemia due to flushing, renal impairment, and mechanical injury of the coronary artery. However, serious complications are rare, and so far intracoronary OFDI imaging is considered safe.[20,21]

13.3   IMAGING PROCEDURE

In the FD-OCT intravascular imaging system, the image is collected from pullback using a nonocclusive technique. The procedures of both FD-OCT types are almost the same, except for purging the catheter sheath with contrast media.

1. A guiding catheter (6 Fr size) is introduced into the ostium of the vessel of interest. In some cases, a 7 Fr system may be preferred. The guiding catheter with a side hall is not recommended.
2. Like with IVUS, the current OCT system requires that the patient is anticoagulated, and typically 30–40 IU/kg (2000–3000 IU) heparin is administered according to the patient's anticoagulation status. The administration of intracoronary nitroglycerin before OCT catheter advance is recommended to minimize the potential for catheter-induced vasospasm.
3. A standard guidewire is passed into the target image vessel distal to the region of interest.
4. The probe interface unit is placed in a sterile sheath, and the OCT catheter is carefully removed from its protective sheath.
5. This step is required for only the OCT catheter produced by St. Jude Medical. The catheter's lumen has to be purged by injection of 1–2 mL of pure contrast before introduction of the catheter into the patient. Flush until three to five drops exit from the catheter's distal tip. This is to ensure that the refractive indexes inside and outside the catheter match.
6. The catheter is connected to the probe interface unit. The catheter is calibrated automatically (Z-offset) but may need manual adjustment. The four calibration markers should be aligned to the outside of the catheter, not to the outside of the fiber optic.
7. Insert the OCT catheter through the guidewire into the coronary artery and advance to the lesion of interest. This procedure should be performed carefully so as not to injure the coronary artery lumen. To ensure successful imaging, keep the OCT catheter and imaging interface in a straight line during imaging acquisition.
8. Start flushing contrast media from the guiding catheter. After a clear view is achieved, immediately begin OCT pullback.

TABLE 13.1
Flush parameters; recommended injection pump settings

Vessel	Flow (mL/S)	Pressure (psi)	Total Volume (mL)
LCA	4	300	14
RCA	3–3.5	300	12–14

Note: LCA, left coronary artery; RCA, right coronary artery.

13.4 FLUSHING PARAMETERS: RECOMMENDED INJECTION SETTING

The appropriate flow rate, pressure, and total volume of flushing media are shown in Table 13.1. As shown below, there are some matters to be attended to perform flushing for each coronary artery.

1. Left anterior descending artery: Standard percutaneous coronary intervention (PCI) guide catheter orientation is typically sufficient.
2. Left circumflex artery: May require guide catheter angle adjustment (rotate the catheter counterclockwise and hold it), or selective engagement to achieve good contrast flow and optimal clearance.
3. Right coronary artery: Adjust contrast injection rate based on the artery diameter. For a small right coronary artery, 3.0 mL/s (total volume 12 mL) may be adequate. However, a large vessel may require 3.5 or 4.0 mL/s (total volume 14 mL).
4. Injection is terminated immediately in the case of chest pain or arrhythmia.

13.5 PITFALLS AND LIMITATIONS

Although OCT provides detailed information on the coronary artery, there are several pitfalls and limitations. We always have to keep those in mind during OFDI imaging.

13.5.1 Incorrect calibration

Correct calibration of the OCT catheter is indispensable for accurate measurement. Hebsgaard et al. reported that a high incidence of incorrect calibration was found in numerous articles from peer-reviewed journals.[22] According to their results, any degree of incorrect calibration of the OFDI catheter was found in 43% of images in articles, and especially serious incorrect calibration was seen in 16%. Although both current OCT systems provide automated calibrations, sometimes failed automated calibration can happen and manual adjustment is required. Figure 13.1 demonstrates a representative case with incorrect calibration. In this kind of case, PCI operators might misjudge the optimal balloon and stent size, which can lead to miserable situations, such as coronary artery dissection and perforation. It is suggested that we always pay careful attention to the correct calibration of the OCT catheter—every time. In addition, after performing OCT imaging and pulling the catheter away from the coronary artery, the calibration will not be correct for the next time session. Therefore, calibration should be done at the next imaging session.

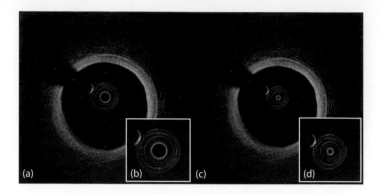

Figure 13.1 Representative case with incorrect calibration. (a) The OCT image at the reference site demonstrates the lumen diameter of the coronary artery (3.43 × 3.57 mm), suggesting the optimal stent size is 3.5 mm. (b) The calibration was incorrect. (c) After the calibration was corrected, the lumen diameter was 3.12 × 3.25 mm and the proper stent size seemed to be 3.25 mm. (d) The calibration was properly adjusted.

13.5.2 Correction with refractive index

To achieve clear imaging, we need to exclude red blood cells from the coronary artery. Although contrast media is widely used for this purpose, an increased total amount of contrast media for OCT imaging acquisition may lead to impairment of renal function, which is called "contrast media–induced nephropathy" (CIN).[23,24] It is recommended that we refrain from higher dose of contrast media, and using an alternative flushing media is one solution for this problem.

According to the fluid dynamics theory, the fluid in a tube can be successfully displaced by the injection of another fluid that has higher viscosity. This phenomenon has been applied to clear blood for intracoronary OCT imaging.[25] Because typical contrast media have a higher viscosity than other solutions, including saline or lactated Ringer's solution, they are appropriate for superior blood displacement, and therefore often chosen for intravascular OCT imaging. Low-molecular-weight dextran L (LMD-L) and a mixture of contrast media and saline (typically 1:1) are also used as alternatives. Studies have revealed that the quality of OCT image acquisition with these flushing media is acceptable and makes it possible to reduce the total amount of contrast media without loss of image quality.[26–28]

The refractive index is a dimensionless number that describes how light propagates through a medium. For example, the refractive index of air is 1.00029, and that of water is 1.3334. Compared with air, light propagates slower in the flushing media or tissues; therefore, measurement data from an OCT image have to be corrected by the refractive index of the flushing solution. Both OCT systems provide a method for correcting measurement data with refractive indexes representative of the flushing media. As shown in Figure 13.2, if not corrected with an appropriate refractive index, the measurement data might be misunderstood, leading to misuse of optimized sizes of the stent or balloon. We have to make sure that measurement data are corrected by the right refractive index.

13.5.3 Filling of catheter sheath with contrast media

The OCT catheter manufactured from St. Jude Medical (St. Paul, Minnesota), the Dragonfly, has a sheath-type structure at the peripheral site of the image core, which has to be filled with pure contrast media before OCT imaging. Incomplete purging of blood from the OCT catheter sheath is also one of the major artifacts that can affect the acquisition of clear OCT images. Contamination of blood or bubbles can disturb visualization of the coronary arteries and affect measurement of data behind those substances (Figure 13.3).

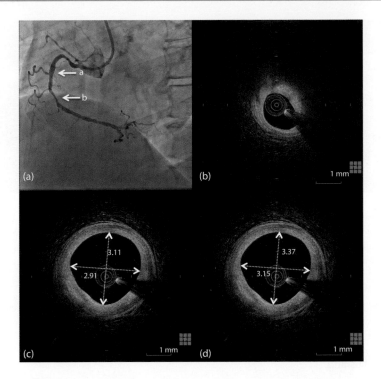

Figure 13.2 Correction with refractive index. An angiography and corresponding OCT image of a patient with stable angina (a–c). Correction with the appropriate refractive index is important to gain accurate measurement data. In this case, intracoronary flushing was done by lactated Ringer's solution and measurement data were corrected by refractive index of lactated Ringer's solution (1.334). The diameters of the coronary artery lumen at the proximal site were 3.11 and 2.91 mm (c). However, if not corrected properly and, for example, corrected by the refractive index of contrast media (1.443), the diameters of the coronary artery at the proximal site were 3.37 and 3.15 mm (d), which might tempt us to choose a larger-size stent or balloon.

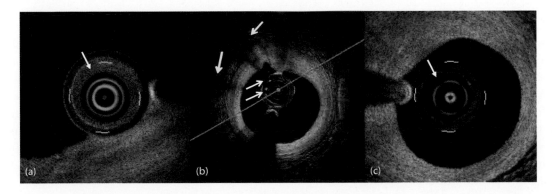

Figure 13.3 Incomplete purge of OCT catheters. (a) Blood in catheter (white arrow). (b) Bubbles in catheter (white arrow) cause OCT signal attenuations (white arrow). (c) Purge good (white arrow).

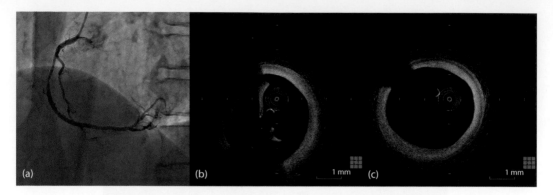

Figure 13.4 Representative case with inadequate flushing. (a) The angiography demonstrates the moderate stenosis at the midportion of the right coronary artery. (b) To evaluate the lesion, OCT was performed, but the lesion was not fully assessed because blood flow attenuated the OCT signals due to inadequate flushing. (c) In this case, the flushing rate was changed from 3.0 to 3.5 mL/s and a clear OCT image session was achieved.

Operators have to make sure the purge is complete and use "pure contrast media," because contrast media can be easily mixed with blood during the procedure.

13.5.4 Inadequate flushing

As red blood cells could attenuate near-infrared light, we have to clear blood flow from the imaging field of view. To acquire OCT imaging, continuous flushing of liquid solutions (contrast media is mainly recommended) from the guiding catheter is currently performed. The appropriate flow rate, pressure, and total volume of flushing media are shown in Table 13.1. This is the default setting, and if a clear OCT image is not acquired, we have to adjust the flushing settings. A higher flow rate and amount of flushing media may be required when using solutions with less viscosity (for example, lactated Ringer's solution or saline) than the contrast media. In addition, we have to confirm whether the guiding catheter is located coaxially for the coronary artery. A guiding catheter with a side hall is not recommended for OCT imaging. Figure 13.4 demonstrates a case with inadequate flushing. In this case, a clear OCT image was achieved after adjusting the flushing rate.

13.5.5 Lesion selection

Lesions with rich collateral blood flow and coronary ostium lesions are not feasible because complete blood clearance is inadequate. If interventional cardiologists need an intracoronary imaging device for coronary intervention in such a case, IVUS-guided PCI might be a better choice.

Also, in lesions with subtotal occlusion, flushing for OCT imaging might not be suitable. Because the profile of current OCT catheters is relatively tight (2.6 or 2.7 Fr diameter) for the coronary vessel lumen, the OCT catheter itself has the potential to disturb flushing flow and/or easily get stuck at the stenotic site. The restoration of antegrade blood flow is recommended prior to OCT examination of that artery. Figure 13.5 demonstrates a representative case with long and severe stenotic lesions, in which a clear OCT image was not achieved before coronary stenting.

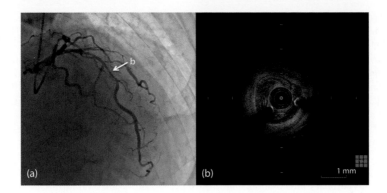

Figure 13.5 Case with severe and long lesion. (a) The coronary angiogram demonstrates the relatively severe and long stenotic lesion at the proximal and midportion of the left anterior descending artery. (b) The OCT image is unclear due to insufficient flushing before coronary intervention.

13.6 CONCLUSIONS

OCT can provide us detailed information and let us make better decisions for coronary therapeutic intervention. However, incorrect assessments and information potentially lead us to make the wrong decisions. At any time while using an OCT system for coronary imaging, operators have to pay careful attention to avoid complications and pitfalls.

REFERENCES

1. Bouma BE, Tearney GJ. Power-efficient nonreciprocal interferometer and linear-scanning fiber-optic catheter for optical coherence tomography. *Optics Letters* 1999;24(8):531–3.
2. Huang D et al. Optical coherence tomography. *Science* 1991;254:1178–81.
3. Jang IK et al. Visualization of coronary atherosclerotic plaques in patients using optical coherence tomography: Comparison with intravascular ultrasound. *Journal of the American College of Cardiology* 2002;39(4):604–9.
4. Brezinski ME et al. Optical coherence tomography for optical biopsy. Properties and demonstration of vascular pathology. *Circulation* 1996;93:1206–13.
5. Jang IK et al. In vivo characterization of coronary atherosclerotic plaque by use of optical coherence tomography. *Circulation* 2005;111(12):1551–5.
6. Kubo T et al. Assessment of culprit lesion morphology in acute myocardial infarction: Ability of optical coherence tomography compared with intravascular ultrasound and coronary angioscopy. *Journal of the American College of Cardiology* 2007;50:933–9.
7. Virmani R et al. Pathology of the vulnerable plaque. *Journal of the American College of Cardiology* 2006;47:C13–8.
8. Bouma BE et al. Evaluation of intracoronary stenting by intravascular optical coherence tomography. *Heart* 2003;89:317–20.
9. Sawada T et al. Persistent malapposition after implantation of sirolimus-eluting stent into intramural coronary hematoma: Optical coherence tomography observations. *Circulation Journal* 2006;70:1515–9.
10. Matsumoto D et al. Neointimal coverage of sirolimus-eluting stents at 6-month follow-up: Evaluated by optical coherence tomography. *European Heart Journal* 2007;28:961–7.
11. Serruys PW et al. Evaluation of the second generation of a bioresorbable everolimus-eluting vascular scaffold for the treatment of de novo coronary artery stenosis: 12-month clinical and imaging outcomes. *Journal of the American College of Cardiology* 2011;58:1578–88.

12. Bourantas CV et al. Effect of the endothelial shear stress patterns on neointimal proliferation following drug-eluting bioresorbable vascular scaffold implantation: An optical coherence tomography study. *JACC Cardiovascular Interventions* 2014;7:315–24.

13. Waksman R et al. Serial observation of drug-eluting absorbable metal scaffold: Multi-imaging modality assessment. *Circulation Cardiovascular Interventions* 2013;6:644–53.

14. Yun SH et al. Comprehensive volumetric optical microscopy in vivo. *Nature Medicine* 2006;12:1429–33.

15. Tearney GJ et al. Three-dimensional coronary artery microscopy by intracoronary optical frequency domain imaging. *JACC Cardiovascular Imaging* 2008;1:752–61.

16. Burzotta F et al. Fractional flow reserve or optical coherence tomography guidance to revascularize intermediate coronary stenosis using angioplasty (FORZA) trial: Study protocol for a randomized controlled trial. *Trials* 2014;15:140.

17. Prati F et al. Angiography alone versus angiography plus optical coherence tomography to guide decision-making during percutaneous coronary intervention: The Centro per la Lotta contro l'Infarto-Optimisation of Percutaneous Coronary Intervention (CLI-OPCI) study. *EuroIntervention* 2012;8:823–9.

18. Prati F et al. Expert's OCT review document. Expert review document on methodology, terminology, and clinical applications of optical coherence tomography: Physical principles, methodology of image acquisition, and clinical application for assessment of coronary arteries and atherosclerosis. *European Heart Journal* 2010;31:401–15.

19. Kataiwa H et al. Head to head comparison between the conventional balloon occlusion method and the non-occlusion method for optical coherence tomography. *International Journal of Cardiology* 2011;146:186–90.

20. Lehtinen T et al. Feasibility and safety of frequency-domain optical coherence tomography for coronary artery evaluation: A single-center study. *International Journal of Cardiovascular Imaging* 2013;29:997–1005.

21. Imola F et al. Safety and feasibility of frequency domain optical coherence tomography to guide decision making in percutaneous coronary intervention. *EuroIntervention* 2010;6:575–81.

22. Hebsgaard L et al. Calibration of intravascular optical coherence tomography as presented in peer reviewed publications. *International Journal of Cardiology* 2014;171:92–3.

23. McCullough PA et al. Acute renal failure after coronary intervention: Incidence, risk factors, and relationship to mortality. *American Journal of Medicine* 1997;103:368–75.

24. Rihal CS et al. Incidence and prognostic importance of acute renal failure after percutaneous coronary intervention. *Circulation* 2002;105:2259–64.

25. Petitjeans P, Maxworthy T. Miscible displacements in capillary tubes. Part 1. Experiments. *Journal of Fluid Mechanics* 1996;326:37–56.

26. Frick K et al. Low molecular weight dextran provides similar optical coherence tomography coronary imaging compared to radiographic contrast media. *Catheterization and Cardiovascular Interventions* 2014;84:727–31.

27. Ozaki Y et al. Comparison of contrast media and low-molecular-weight dextran for frequency-domain optical coherence tomography. *Circulation Journal* 2012;76:922–7.

28. Li X et al. Safety and efficacy of frequency domain optical coherence tomography in pigs. *EuroIntervention* 2011;7:497–504.

Appendix: Intravascular Bioresorbable Vascular Scaffold Optimization Technique

Jun Li and Hiram Bezerra

The Food and Drug Administration approval of Absorb GT1 (Abbott Vascular, Santa Clara, CA), the first generation bioresorbable vascular scaffold (BVS) for use in the coronaries, was unfortunately met soon by concerns of scaffold thrombosis at a higher rate when compared to best-in-class drug-eluting stent (DES).[1-3] From this early experience we have learned the importance of proper scaffold implantation technique to minimize device failure.[4] The implantation technique currently advocated involves proper lesion preparation, sizing, and postdilation (PSP).

In our experience, intravascular imaging is an integral extension of the PSP technique. Although both intravascular ultrasound (IVUS) and optical coherence tomography (OCT) will provide information on target lesion diameter, tissue characterization, and landing zone suitability, there are important differences to consider. Specifically, the limitations of IVUS in BVS implantation include: inability to discern calcium depth, achieve precise longitudinal analysis, and inadequate evaluation of scaffold strut apposition after implantation. Given these shortcomings, OCT is our preferred modality of intravascular imaging to guide BVS implantation. Our protocol for intravascular BVS Optimization Technique (iBOT) is detailed below.

iBOT

Our BVS implantation strategy (Figure A.1) hinges on the use of imaging before and after scaffold implantation for procedural planning, preparation, sizing, postdilation, and optimization. Pre-implantation imaging is particularly important for determination of the degree of calcification to assess the need for atherectomy, and appropriate scaffold sizing.

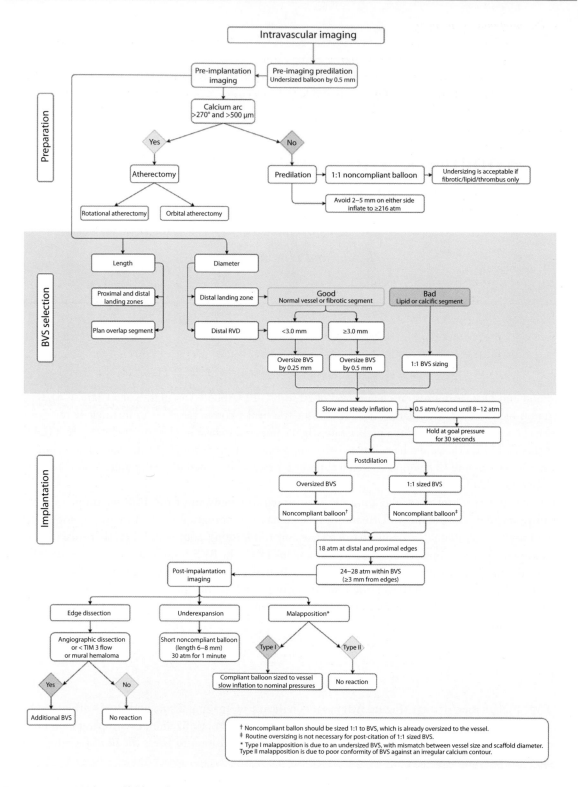

Figure A.1 iBOT for scaffold implantation.

I. *Pre-implantation imaging.*

  A. Predilation with a balloon *undersized by 0.5 mm* (based on angiographic assessment) to achieve ample lumen size for intravascular imaging catheter.

  B. Intravascular imaging to determine degree and depth of calcification, proximal and distal reference vessel diameter (RVD), and lesion length. Decision making based on each component is further discussed.

II. *Lesion preparation.*

  A. *Balloon predilation.* Use 1:1 sized, noncompliant balloon for predilation, achieving good expansion of the balloon. This may require balloon pressures of 16 atmospheres (atm).

    1. Avoid 2–5 mm on the intended proximal and distal landing zones.

    2. Undersized predilation balloons may be sufficient in lesions with soft composition (e.g., fibro-lipidic plaque or thrombotic lesions).

    3. Scoring balloons may be indicated for concentric, fibro-calcified plaques with calcium burden that do not reach the atherectomy threshold.

  B. *Atherectomy.*

    1. *Calcium.* In lesions with calcium arc >270° and >500 μm in thickness,[9] either rotational or orbital atherectomy is recommended for calcium modification and debulking. In the absence of thick circumferential calcium, balloon predilation is usually adequate to achieve the necessary luminal gain (Figure A.2).

    2. *In-stent restenosis (ISR).* The majority of lesions within previous stents tend to have fibrotic tissue buildup, consistent with neointimal hyperplasia (NIH). A fraction of ISR will be secondary to neoatherosclerosis, characterized by lipid and/or calcium deposits seen on OCT (Figure A.3). Seldomly, microvasculature may also be seen within a segment of neoatherosclerosis. In the absence of a technical mechanism for stent failure (e.g., underexpansion of previous stent), BVS may be useful as a means to deliver antiproliferative drugs without leaving an additional metallic stent.

      a. *NIH.* Laser atherectomy can be utilized to help modify the fibrotic tissue. Scoring balloons may be a useful adjunct to achieve sufficient luminal gain prior to BVS implantation (Figure A.4).

      b. *Neoatherosclerosis.* Adequate predilation can typically be performed with a noncompliant balloon sized 1:1 to previous stent.

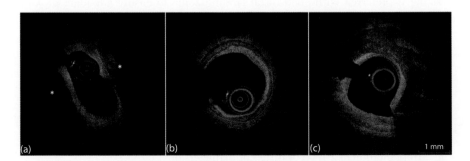

Figure A.2 A spectrum of calcifications as seen on OCT. Panel (a) shows two distinct, thick calcific nodules (asterisks) separated by fibrotic tissue. Panel (b) shows thin, circumferential calcification. Panel (c) shows calcium arc >270° with a thickness of 800 μm. The lesion in panel (c) will necessitate atherectomy for adequate luminal gain.

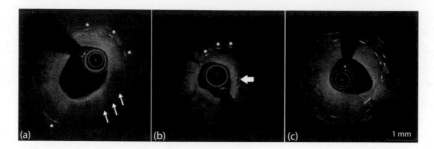

Figure A.3 Examples of types of in-stent restenosis. Panels (a) and (b) show evidence of neoatheroclerosis. The asterisks indicate the presence of a previous metallic stent. Narrow arrows highlight the presence of lipid within the in-stent restenosis, while the broad arrow shows the presence of microvasculature. Both of these findings are consistent with neoatherosclerosis. Panel (c) shows the presence of three layers of metallic stent, with fibrotic tissue consistent with neointimal hyperplasia.

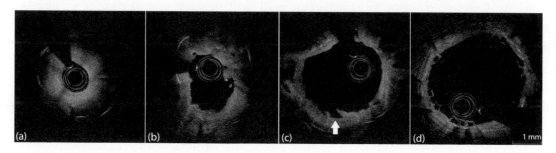

Figure A.4 A patient with severe in-stent restenosis of a prior right coronary artery DES. Panel (a) shows the fulminant fibrotic, neointimal hyperplasia. Panel (b) shows the tissue ablation achieved following laser atherectomy with a 0.9 mm catheter at rate and fluency of 80 and 80. Panel (c) shows the luminal gain achieved with a subsequent scoring balloon with a diameter of 3.0 mm. Broad arrow marks an imprint created by the scoring balloon. Panel (d) shows the deployment of a BVS with a diameter of 3.0 mm; note the minimal residual tissue between the prior metallic stent and the new BVS.

III. *BVS selection.*

    A. *Diameter.* The BVS diameter is dictated by the distal landing zone quality and RVD (Figure A.5). Oversizing is preferred with good distal landing zones to ensure adequate proximal scaffold apposition.

        1. Good distal landing zone quality (i.e., normal vessel or fibrotic only lesion):

            a. If distal RVD <3.0 mm, then oversize BVS by 0.25 mm.

            b. If distal RVD ≥3.0 mm, then oversize BVS by 0.5 mm.

        2. Bad distal landing zone quality (i.e., eccentric calcium or lipid lesion):

            a. BVS sized 1:1 based on the distal RVD.

        3. With significant vessel tapering (>1.0 mm) between the proximal and distal landing zones, the operator should consider either:

            a. Implantation of 2 BVS of different diameters or

            b. Implantation of a metallic stent.

    This is in an effort to avoid scaffold malapposition due to an undersized BVS in the proximal segment.

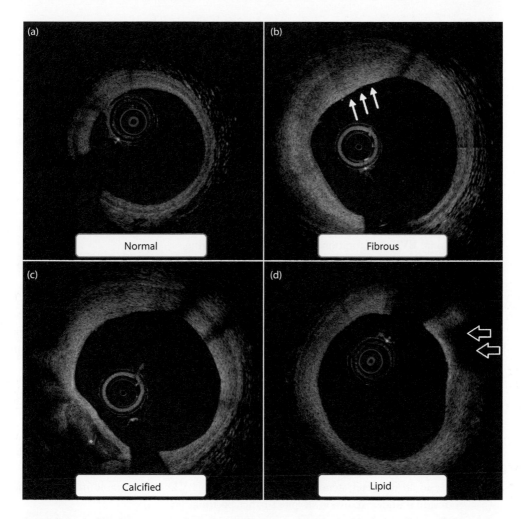

Figure A.5 A reference of landing zone qualities. Panel (a) shows a normal vessel with three layers of the vessel wall present (intima, media, and adventitia). Panel (b) shows a fibrotic lesion (narrow arrows). Panel (c) shows a calcific nodule (asterisk), while panel (d) shows a lipid rich lesion (hollow arrows). While distal landing zones that correspond to panels (a) and (b) may receive an oversized BVS as outlined, in the distal landing zones akin to panels (c) and (d), the BVS should be 1:1 sized.

 B. *Length.*
  1. If >1 BVS is required, the planned overlap segment should be free of severe disease if possible.
  2. The integrated lumen profile with volumetric analysis on OCT is helpful in planning for scaffold length. OCT provides a distinct advantage over IVUS for accurate length determination, as previously discussed.
IV. *Scaffold implantation.*
 A. Slow and steady deployment, inflating approximately 0.5 atm per second until 8–12 atm.
  1. The goal pressure should be maintained for a minimum of 30 seconds.
 B. Implantation of 2 sequential scaffolds should minimize overlapping struts.
  1. The distal balloon marker of the more proximal, undeployed BVS should be touching or "kissing" the scaffold marker of the more distal, implanted BVS.

V. *Postdilation.*
  A. Noncompliant balloons, sized 1:1 to the scaffold, should be used for postdilation.
     1. High pressures of 24–28 atm should be used within the BVS (≥3 mm from edges).
     2. Lower pressures (e.g., approximately 18 atm) should be used at the edges.
  B. Routine oversizing of the postdilation balloon is not necessary.
     1. If vessel tapering is present, the proximal and middle segments of the BVS should be post-dilated with a short, noncompliant balloon with a diameter sized to the proximal RVD.
  C. Stent optimization tools (e.g., stent boost) should be utilized when available to ensure positioning of the postdilation balloons within the scaffold.
VI. *Post-implantation imaging.*
  A. Intravascular imaging is performed after postdilation to assess for edge dissection, underexpansion, and malapposition of the BVS.
     1. *Edge dissection.* If an edge dissection is seen on intravascular imaging, the decision for an additional BVS implantation depends on the following.
        a. In the presence of a normal angiogram (no dissection, preservation of TIMI 3 flow), no further intervention is needed.
        b. In the presence of a concurrent mural hematoma on intravascular imaging, an additional scaffold is necessary to cover the dissection, even in the presence of a normal angiogram.
     2. *Expansion.* Underexpansion is the result of cross-sectional luminal areas that are smaller than the RVD. The lumen profile and volumetric analysis obtained via OCT are useful instruments to help identify areas of underexpansion (Figure A.6).
        a. Underexpanded segments should be further postdilated.
           i. Typically, short (6–8 mm), noncompliant balloons at high pressures of 30 atm for at least 1 minute are adequate to achieve better expansion.
           ii. Additional oversizing (0.25 mm) of the postdilation noncompliant balloon can be considered. However, this is not recommended in regions with eccentric calcium due to the risk of vessel rupture.
        b. Residual diameter stenosis ≤15% compared to RVD is acceptable in the presence of residual underexpansion despite further postdilation.

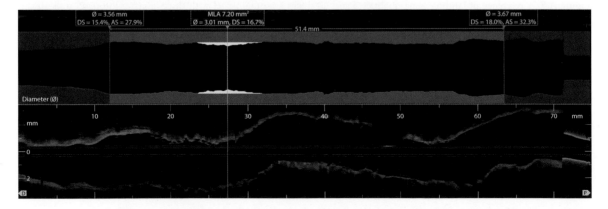

Figure A.6 A volumetric analysis (top panel) and lumen profile (bottom panel) showing an area of scaffold underexpansion, as highlighted by yellow. This appears as a waist in the volumetric analysis. Further high-pressure postdilation is recommended at the underexpanded segment.

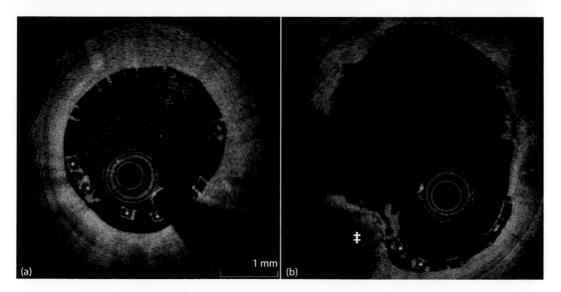

Figure A.7 Two types of malapposition, with malapposed struts highlighted by asterisks. Panel (a) shows type I malapposition, in which there is a scaffold-vessel wall size mismatch. This can be alleviated by slow inflation of a compliant balloon sized 1:1 to the vessel wall, up to nominal pressures. Panel (b) shows type II malapposition, the result of a protruding calcium nodule (‡) resulting in nonconformity of the strut against the irregular vessel wall contour. This should not be aggressively postdilated.

3. *Apposition*. Malapposition is defined as a lack of contact between the scaffold struts and the vessel wall. Two types of malapposition can occur.
   a. Type I: undersized scaffold, creating a mismatch between vessel size and scaffold diameter (Figure A.7a).
      i. This can be alleviated with further postdilation with a compliant balloon, sized 1:1 to the RVD. The balloon should be slowly inflated to nominal pressures to allow scaffold growth.
   b. Type II: nonconformity of BVS to a vessel wall due to irregular calcium contour (Figure A.7b).
      i. This does not need to be aggressively corrected. Rather, the focus should be on ensuring adequate lumen expansion as previously discussed.

REFERENCES

1. Lipinski MJ et al. Scaffold thrombosis after percutaneous coronary intervention with ABSORB Bioresorbable Vascular Scaffold: A systematic review and meta-analysis. *JACC Cardiovascular Interventions* 2016;9:12–24.
2. Collet C et al. Late thrombotic events after bioresorbable scaffold implantation: A systematic review and meta-analysis of randomized clinical trials. *European Heart Journal* 2017.
3. Ellis SG. Everolimus-eluting bioresorbable vascular scaffolds in patients with coronary artery disease: ABSORB III trial 2-year results. *ACC 2017*. March 18, 2017.
4. "Simple PSP implant strategy." *Absorb GT1, Abbott Vascular*. 2017.
5. Gutierrez-Chico JL et al. Quantitative multi-modality imaging analysis of a fully bioresorbable stent: A head-to-head comparison between QCA, IVUS and OCT. *International Journal of Cardiovascular Imaging* 2012;28:467–78.

6. Negi SI, Rosales O. The role of intravascular optical coherence tomography in peripheral percutaneous interventions. *Journal of Invasive Cardiology* 2013;25:E51–3.

7. Bezerra HG et al. Optical coherence tomography versus intravascular ultrasound to evaluate coronary artery disease and percutaneous coronary intervention. *JACC Cardiovascular Interventions* 2013;6:228–36.

8. Tenekecioglu E et al. Intracoronary optical coherence tomography: Clinical and research applications and intravascular imaging software overview. *Catheterization and Cardiovascular Interventions* 2017.

9. Maejima N et al. Relationship between thickness of calcium on optical coherence tomography and crack formation after balloon dilatation in calcified plaque requiring rotational atherectomy. *Circulation Journal* 2016;80:1413–9.

10. Pighi M et al. Imaging and functional assessment of bioresorbable scaffolds. *Minerva Cardioangiologica* 2016;64:442–61.

Index

A

ABSORB II trial, 141
Absorb GT, 189
Acute coronary syndrome (ACS), 7, 97
Angio coregistration software, 158–160, 168
Angiotensin-converting-enzyme (ACE) inhibitors, 47
Apposition, 190, 195
Atherectomy, 190, 191
Atherosclerotic SCAD (A-SCAD), 98

B

Balloon angioplasty (BA), 43
    cutting, 130
    drug-eluting, 29
    focal force, 131
    percutaneous, 90
    plain old, 46
    scoring, 30
Balloon predilation, 190, 191
Bare-metal stent (BMS), 14, 30, 46
Bioresorbable vascular scaffolds (BVSs), 135–143, 181
    diameter, 192, 193
    follow-up, OCT assessment for, 139–142
    length, 193
    implantation, OCT assessment after, 138–139
    implantation, OCT assessment before, 136–138
    implantation in calcified plaque, 137
    measurement of scaffold area, 139
    optimization technique, intravascular, see Intravascular Bioresorbable vascular scaffold optimization technique (iBOT)
    overlapped segments, 139
    platform components, 135
    selection, 190, 192–193
    "vascular restoration therapy," 135
BMS, see Bare-metal stent (BMS)

C

CAD, *see* Coronary artery disease (CAD)
Calcium, 60, 190, 191, 193, 195
Canadian Cardiovascular Society (CCS) III angina, 89
Cardiac allograft vasculopathy (CAV) after heart transplantation, 111–121
  atherosclerotic plaques, 116–118
  background, 111
  cellular rejection, 118
  intimal hyperplasia, 115–116
  IVUS and, 118
  neovascularization, 118
  OCT utilization post–heart transplantation, 115–118
  pathophysiology, 112–115
  plaque rupture, 118
  rejection, 114–115
  risk factors, 113
  screening and diagnosis, 112
  traditional atherosclerosis, 115
  treatment, 119
CB, *see* Cutting balloon (CB)
Celiac disease, 98
Chronic total occlusion (CTO), 132, 141
Churg–Strauss syndrome, 98
CMV, *see* Cytomegalovirus (CMV)
Computed tomography angiography (CTA), 112
Contrast media–induced nephropathy (CIN), 184
Coronary arteries, OCT assessment out of, 123–134
  angioplasty, 130
  assessment of interventional techniques, 130–132
  atherectomy, 132
  clinical applications of OCT in peripheral vasculature, 126–132
  color flow and three-dimensional reconstruction, 124
  future directions, 132–133
  history of intravascular imaging, 123–124
  IVUS, 124–125
  lesion characterization, 127–130
  lumen profile, 129
  optical coherence tomography, 124–126
  stent, 132
  technique, 125–126
Coronary artery disease (CAD), 1, 115
Cutting balloon (CB), 30, 43
  calcium modification using, 60
  case, 130
  dilatation device, 44
Cutting Balloon Global Randomized Trial, 45
Cutting and scoring plaque pretreatment, *see* Plaque modification
Cytomegalovirus (CMV), 112

D

Data acquisition system (DAS), 150
Dragonfly (catheter), 184
Driver-motor and optical controller (DOC), 148
Drug-eluting balloons (DEBs), 29

Drug-eluting stent (DES), 2
    alternative to, 135
    challenges, 30
    neoatherosclerotic changes in, 86
    stent expansion and, 43
BVS and, 189

E

Edge dissection, 190, 194
Ehler–Danlos syndrome type 4, 98
Electro-optical (EO) circuit, 150
Everolimus-eluting stents (EESs), 65, 78
Expansion, post-implantation imaging, 190, 194
External elastic membrane (EEM), 10, 14
External iliac artery (EIA), 130

F

FastView imaging catheter, 163–166
    characteristics, 165–166
    clinical setup and compatibility, 163–165
    components and architecture, 163
    dimensions, 165
FFR technology, *see* Fractional flow reserve (FFR) technology
Fibromuscular dysplasia (FMD), 98, 99–100
Fourier-domain OCT (FD-OCT), 146; *see also* Left main assessment
    frequency swept, 125
    ILUMIEN OPTIS and OPTIS, 146
    imaging speeds, 146
    operating principles, 146
    systems, 3, 21
Fractional flow reserve (FFR) technology, 145

G

Geographic miss, 70, 81, 87
Giant cell arteritis, 98

I

iBOT, *see* Intravascular Bioresorbable vascular scaffold optimization technique (iBOT)
ILUMIEN OPTIS Mobile and OPTIS Integrated System overview, 125, 145–161
    Angio coregistration software, 158–160
    catheter specifications, 147–148
    comparison of specs, 148
    FD-OCT operating principles, 146
    ILUMIEN OPTIS Mobile System, 148–150
    low coherence interferometry, 146
    OCT application software, 155–158
    OPTIS Integrated System, 150–154
    platform overview, 145–148
    system specifications, 146
Imaging acquisition, *see* OCT imaging acquisition
Implantation, scaffold, 190, 193
In-stent restenosis (ISR), 14, 30 191, 192

Intramural hematoma (IMH), 98, 106
Intravascular Bioresorbable vascular scaffold optimization technique (iBOT), 189–196
    overview, 189, 190
    pre-implantation imaging, 190, 191
    lesion preparation, 190, 191, 192
    BVS selection, 190, 192–193
    scaffold implantation, 190, 193
    postdilation, 190, 194
    post-implantation imaging, 190, 194–195
Intravascular ultrasound (IVUS), 1, 46, 59
    -CBA-BMS, 46
    cutoff value, 71
    detection of CAV by, 112
    efficacy of during PCI, 75
    -guided high-pressure balloon postdilatation, 1
    introduction of, 123
    OCT compared with, 136
    study of late ST using, 92
    traditional use of, 29
ISR, *see* In-stent restenosis (ISR)
IVUS, *see* Intravascular ultrasound (IVUS)

K

Kawasaki, 98
Kissing balloon inflation (KBT), 67, 78

L

LAD, *see* Left anterior descendent artery (LAD)
Landing zones, 192, 193
Late stent failure, 85–95
    case report (in-stent restenosis), 89–90
    distal edge restenosis, 88
    intrastent pathology, 92–93
    lipid-rich in-stent plaque, 87
    neointima, 86
    OCT guide therapy, 93–94
    restenosis, 85–89
    stent thrombosis, 91–94
    stent underexpansion, 88
Left anterior descendent artery (LAD), 9, 30, 89
Left circumflex artery (LCX), 89
Left main assessment, 75–83
    angiographic characteristics, 76
    FD-OCT measurements for ULM disease, 77–78
    feasibility of FD-OCT for ULM disease, 78–82
    imagine procedure characteristics, 77
    kissing balloon inflation, 78, 81
    malapposed stent struts, 80
    safety of FD-OCT for ULM disease, 75–77
Lesion preparation, 190, 191, 192
Loeys–Dietz syndrome, 98
Low-coherence interferometry, 146
Low-molecular-weight dextran L (LMD-L), 184

LUNAWAVE OFDI imaging console, 166–172
    evaluation of bifurcation lesion, 170–172
    file export, 172
    image acquisition setups, 167–168
    laser safety mechanisms, 166
    PCI procedure evaluation, 169–170
    polygon scanner wavelength filter, 166
    reliability, 167
    sensitivity peak shift, 166
    stent implantation supporting software, 168

M

Magnetic resonance imaging (MRI), 112
Major adverse cardiac events (MACEs), 59, 69
Malapposition, 190, 195
Marfan's syndrome, 98
MI, *see* Myocardial infarction (MI)
Minimal lumen area (MLA), 3
Minimal lumen diameters (MLDs), 4
Minimum stent area (MSA), 46
Minimum stent diameter (MSD), 46
MRI, *see* Magnetic resonance imaging (MRI)
Myocardial infarction (MI), 1

N

Neoartherosclerosis, 191, 192
Neointimal hyperplasia (NIH), 191, 192
Noncompliant (NC) balloon, 30
Non-ST-elevation myocardial infarction (NSTEMI), 7, 30
Nonuniform rotational distortions (NURDs), 165

O

OCT, *see* Optical coherence tomography (OCT)
OCT imaging acquisition, 181–188
    contrast media–induced nephropathy, 184
    correction with refractive index, 184
    filling of catheter sheath with contrast media, 184–186
    flushing parameters (recommended injection setting), 183
    imaging procedure, 182
    inadequate flushing, 186
    incorrect calibration, 183
    lesion selection, 186–187
    pitfalls and limitations, 183–187
    system of OCT, 181–182
    vulnerable plaques, 181
OFDI, *see* Optical frequency-domain imaging (OFDI)
Optical coherence tomography (OCT), 181
    evaluation of intracoronary stents using, 85
    intracoronary, 181
    luminal information provided by, 59
    in plaque pretreatment, 43
    role of in guiding PCI, 75

Optical frequency-domain imaging (OFDI), 181; *see also* Terumo OFDI system
OPTIS Integrated System, 125; *see also* ILUMIEN OPTIS Mobile and OPTIS Integrated System overview

P

PAD, *see* Peripheral arterial disease (PAD)
Percutaneous balloon angioplasty (PTCA), 45
Percutaneous coronary intervention (PCI)
    advancements, 1
    basis of, 29
    BVS, 135, 140
    plaque modification and, 43
    second- and third-generation optimization platforms, 145
    of ULM coronary artery disease, 75
Percutaneous transluminal angioplasty (PTA), 130
Peripheral arterial disease (PAD), 123
Plain old balloon angioplasty (POBA), 46
Plaque modification, 43–58
    before coronary artery stenting using cutting/scoring balloon, 43
    clinical cases using cutting and scoring plaque pretreatment, 46–57
    cutting and scoring balloons, 43–44
    LAD/diagonal bifurcation stenosis, 47, 52
    trial results with cutting or scoring balloon plaque pretreatment, 45–46
Plaque modification, assessment of, 29–42
    burr-to-artery ratio, 35
    cavity-type stent edge dissection, 39
    coronary calcified plaques, morphological patterns of, 37
    cutting balloon or scoring balloon angioplasty, 30
    final angiography after PCI, 30
    flap-type dissection, 39
    in-stent restenosis lesions, 32
    plain ordinary balloon and drug-eluting balloon angioplasty, 29–41
    plaque modification after stenting, 39
    rotational atherectomy, 31, 34, 38
    stent edge dissection, 40
    stent–tissue interaction, 41
POBA, *see* Plain old balloon angioplasty (POBA)
Post-implantation imaging, 190, 194–195
    apposition, 190, 195
    edge dissection, 190, 194
    expansion, 190, 194
Predicted stent area (PSA), 46
Predicted stent diameter (PSD), 46
Pre-implantation imaging, 190, 191
PTA, *see* Percutaneous transluminal angioplasty (PTA)
PTCA, *see* Percutaneous balloon angioplasty (PTCA)

Q

Quantitative coronary angiography (QCA), 4, 46

R

RA, *see* Rotational atherectomy (RA)
RCA, *see* Right coronary artery (RCA)
Reference vessel diameter (RVD), 192, 193

Restenosis, 85–89
  distal edge, 88
  in-stent, 32, 89–90
  management, 87–89
  OCT patterns of, 86–87
  pathobiology of, 85
Restenosis Reduction by Cutting Balloon Evaluation III (REDUCE III), 46
Rheumatoid arthritis, 98
Riga bifurcation registry, 45
Right coronary artery (RCA), 9, 31, 40
Rotational atherectomy (RA), 34
  calcium modification using, 60
  lesions treated with, 31
  plaque modification by, 38

S

Scaffold implantation, 193
Scoring balloon catheter, 44
Single-photon emission computed tomography (SPECT), 33
Spectral/Fourier-domain OCT (SD-OCT), 46
Spontaneous coronary artery dissection (SCAD), 97–109
  angiographic features, 100–101
  diagnosis and management, role of OCT in, 102–105
  epidemiology, 97–98
  fibromuscular dysplasia, 99–100
  "full metal jacket," 106
  intracoronary imaging, 102
  management, 105–106
  pathogenesis, 98–99
  PCI, OCT guidance for, 104–105
  precipitating stress events, 98
  stent strut apposition, 104
SS-OCT, see Swept-source OCT (SS-OCT)
ST, see Stent thrombosis (ST)
ST-elevation myocardial infarction (STEMI), 7, 31, 91
Stent boost, 194
Stent failure, see Late stent failure
Stent optimization, 59–73
  ambiguous angiography, 60
  best stent landing zone, defining of, 62
  bifurcation stenting, 64
  calcium modification using rotational atherectomy or cutting balloon, 60
  edge dissection, 69
  geographic miss, 70
  Ilumien Optis lumen profile, 62
  incomplete lesion coverage, 70–71
  lumen profile, defining of, 60–62
  side branch protection, OCT for, 64–72
  stent deployment, OCT after, 65
  stent length and diameter, OCT for defining, 60–63
  stent malapposition, 65–68
  stent underexpansion, 68
  thin-cap fibroatheromas, 63
  thrombectomy, 59–60
  tissue prolapse, 71–72

unstable plaques, screening for, 62
vessel preparation, utilization of OCT for, 59–60
Stent planning, 1–27
acute stent failure, 18
anatomic landmarks and stenosis severity, 4
concepts, 2
coronary stenosis severity, assessment of, 3–5
in-stent dissections, tissue prolapse, and in-stent thrombus, 20–21
lesion morphology, composition, and morphometry (assessment of), 5–9
PCI planning and guidance, potential clinical impact of OCT use for, 21–22
polymeric bioresorbable scaffold, implantation of, 10
postintervention OCT imaging, 14–21
preintervention OCT imaging, 3–14
stent apposition, 16–17
stent edge dissections, 19
stent expansion, 14–16
stent sizing, 12, 15
vessel measurements for stent sizing, 9–14
Stent thrombosis (ST), 85
Swept-source OCT (SS-OCT), 146

T

Target lesion failure (TLF), 141
Target lesion revascularization (TLR), 45
Target vessel revascularization (TVR), 45
TCFA, *see* Thin-cap fibroatheroma (TCFA)
TD-OCT, *see* Time-domain OCT (TD-OCT)
Terumo OFDI system, 163–180
case report (bifurcation PCI), 177–179
case report (separated proximal and mid–left anterior descending artery lesions), 172–177
FastView imaging catheter, 163–166
Lunawave OFDI imaging console, 166–172
Thin-cap fibroatheroma (TCFA), 7, 12, 181
Thrombolysis in myocardial infarction (TIMI), 7, 31, 47, 105
Time-domain OCT (TD-OCT), 3, 124, 146
TLF, *see* Target lesion failure (TLF)
TLR, *see* Target lesion revascularization (TLR)
Type I malapposition, 190, 195
Type II malapposition, 190, 195

U

Unprotected left main (ULM) coronary artery disease, 75; *see also* Left main assessment

V

"Vascular restoration therapy," 135
Vulnerable plaques, 181

W

Wegener granulomatosis, 98

X

X-View mode, 168